Library of Congress Cataloging-in-Publication Data

VanValkenburgh, Nicky.
Train Your Brain, Transform Your Life: Conquer Attention Deficit Hyperactivity Disorder In 60 Days, Without Ritalin.
Nicky VanValkenburgh. – 1st ed.
Includes References.
ISBN 978-0-615-29794-1
1. Attention Deficit Hyperactivity Disorder– Treatment. 2. Neuro-plasticity. 3. Brain Training – Brain Fitness – Rehabilitation.
Library of Congress Control Number: 2010928249

Proofreading by Kalinda Rose Stevenson, David Siever, and Amanda Jackson.

Photograph of the author by Sheryl Renee Duckett, Manna Photographics. www.mannaphotographics.com

Published by Petrie Press.
14 Ingram Blvd. La Vergne, TN 37086

Author's website:
www.TrainYourBrainTransformYourLife.com

Train Your Brain, Transform Your Life:

*Conquer Attention Deficit Hyperactivity Disorder
In 60 Days, Without Ritalin*

By Nicky VanValkenburgh

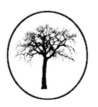

PETRIE PRESS
www.TrainYourBrainTransformYourLife.com

DISCLAIMER AND LEGAL NOTICES

FEEDBACK:
WHAT PEOPLE ARE SAYING ABOUT THIS BOOK

"As an educator, this book's concept of a drug-free, non-evasive approach to ADHD is very appealing to me. I've spent the last 30 years teaching students with ADHD in both public schools and colleges. I'll be recommending the ALERT to my students. In fact, I encourage everyone with ADHD to buy this book. The concept of brain training is a breakthrough for millions of school age children and parents who are looking for a different solution. If you are looking for a natural alternative that doesn't just sedate you, but actually reduces your ADHD symptoms, this book is for you.

"Another thing that I like about *Train Your Brain* is that it is written in a warm, conversational style. It's as if Nicky is sitting next to me in a chair, talking to me. What a difference from books that are cold, clinical and overly complicated. *Train Your Brain* is engaging and easily digested. It demystifies the causes and symptoms of ADHD and will enlighten anyone who struggles with ADHD."

Daria T. Cronic, Ph.D.
Educational Consultant and SIM Professional Developer
Clinton, SC.

"If you're looking for a natural, drug-free way to conquer your ADHD then this book is a gem! It's well-written, organized, provides the facts and lots of smart advice. The approach is different than what I have advocated in my counseling practice, but I think that ALERT brain training is a great idea for increasing a person's concentration, focus and retention. Perhaps it could be used in addition to counseling for maximum effectiveness."

Dr. Kenneth Herman
Clinical Psychologist
Author, *Secrets From The Sofa: A Psychologist's Guide To Personal Peace.*
Wyckoff, NJ.

"I'm delighted that Nicky has written this book about a natural cure for ADHD. If you could see the amount of ADHD drugs that are filled in one day in a pharmacy, it would shock you. I've spent several years working in a pharmacy, and am amazed at how many parents come in and purchase numerous drugs for their kids. Many of these kids look like walking zombies! Their parents grab anything their doctor prescribes, without thinking twice about what they're putting in their children's bodies. It's scary! Working in a pharmacy opened my eyes at how over-medicated our world has become."

Rita Wiggs
Homemaker and mother
Simpsonville, SC.

"This is the finest book that I've come across that applies light and sound technology to ADHD. I've been utilizing light and sound machines for 25 years now, and am excited to see this technology being used to help children and adults conquer ADHD. It is a much better solution than drugs.

"I'm a consultant to manufacturers, distributor of various light and sound machines and publisher of the AVS Journal. Over the years, I have sold hundreds of light and sound machines, and have witnessed firsthand this technology's potential to train your brain and transform your life. This is no exaggeration! I have met people from all walks of life whose lives are changed by light and sound technology: Young and old, educated and uneducated, sick and well, the troubled and mentally stable. I like the way this book explains this technology in a way that is simple, easy to understand, and slightly entertaining. I encourage everyone who has ADHD to read this book, and consider this all-natural, drug free, and life changing approach."

Michael Landgraf
Publisher of the *AVS Journal*.
Consultant to Microfirm, Inc. (Manufacturer of brainwave synchronizer instruments) and OPNET, Inc. (Developers of Neuro Learning)
Author of *Mind States: An Introduction To Light And Sound Technology*.
http://www.Mindmachines.com/
http://www.Brainmachines.com/
Granada Hills, CA.

"*Train Your Brain* tackles the difficult subject of ADHD from the brain's perspective. The recent discovery of the brain's ability to continue to change and build new neurons and repair damaged neurons into old age is revolutionary. I enjoyed reading Nicky's explanation of electro-chemical imbalances in the ADHD brain and how the ALERT can stimulate and arouse the brain with audio-visual technology. If you're interested in a natural way to reduce ADHD, this book is definitely worth reading."

Deborah Merlin
Author, *Victory Over ADHD: A Holistic Approach For Helping Children With Attention Deficit Hyperactivity Disorder.*
www.VictoryOverADHD.com
Los Angeles, CA.

"Nicky Vanvalkenburgh hits a home run with *Train Your Brain.* You'll know within the first few pages that Nicky has walked in the shoes of ADHD. This book offers answers for anyone wanting to leave the frustration of ADHD behind, and start living the life they've always wanted."

Vincent Harris
"America's Body Language Guy"
Author of *Bypassing No In Business.*
www.VinceHarris.com
Trenton, MI.

"This is more than a book, it's a personal testimony from a woman who has conquered ADHD. Nicky empowers others to take control of their ADHD through empathy, passion and practicality. I found this book to interesting and very easy to follow. She provides an alternative to drugs through her ALERT system for training the brain. Very inspiring and insightful. Lives will be transformed!"

Jaime L. Rohadfox
Author, *Give It Up, Turn It Loose: A Woman's Journey From Dominion To Deliverance*
Certified Life Coach for Women
Founder of Women of Divine Aspiration, LLC.
Charlotte, NC.

"*Train Your Brain* is the key to unlocking the secrets to ADHD and ridding your life of its challenges— without drugs, doctors, or drawn out therapies. Instead of Ritalin, the secret to overcoming ADHD lies in understanding your brain and how it functions. No long, complicated, or hard to understand concepts here. Nicky does a great job of making ADHD easy to understand and easy to conquer. Plus, she reveals a strategy for peak performance. Every teacher, parent and grandparent needs to read this book!"

Harlan Goerger
Business Consultant, Coach, Trainer
Author of *The Selling Gap*; *Bypassing No In Business*, and *Business Expert Guide To Business Success*.
www.AskHG.com
Fargo, ND.

"I enjoyed reading *Train Your Brain*, especially chapter 11, which mentions step class. As a group fitness instructor, I've noticed that it takes the average person at least three times to feel comfortable with the step routine. After that, the brain picks up on the cues easily and you don't even think about what's next. The body just reacts and performs. You get a great workout, and it's a lot of fun with the music and moves involved. This book's brain training program embodies the same fitness principle. You practice the Rhythm of Peak Performance until it becomes an automatic response. This makes a lot of sense to me."

Lynette Froehlich
Group Fitness Instructor, Sportsclub Inc.
Ace Certified Personal Trainer
Chi Running Instructor
Racquetball Pro
http://www.MeltDownSC.Blogspot.com
Greenville, SC.

"Nicky has a knack for putting scientific information into layman's terms. I enjoyed reading this book and am using the ALERT."

Dave Weiner
Buffalo Grove, IL.

"Some books are interesting. Some are entertaining. And some books change lives. Nicky VanValkenburgh's book is one of the life changers. She does more than identify the problem of ADHD, she offers a real solution that is simple, effective, and doesn't involve drugs. This book is a unique combination of clearly explained science and the compassion that can come only from someone who knows firsthand how devastating ADHD can be. Nicky tells her story of her life with ADHD and her amazing discovery of the simple light and sound technology that set her free."

Kalinda Rose Stevenson, Ph.D.
Author of Best Books Award Winner, *No Money Limits,* and *Going Broke With Jesus.*
www.NoMoneyLimits.com
Las Vegas, NV.

"My favorite chapters from *Train Your Brain* deal with stress and relaxation. I've read them seven or eight times. I'm a Massage Therapist, and these chapters caused me to think about the clients I see every day. They often talk to me about their conflicts and personal relationships. Their emotional stress is just as dangerous as being out of shape physically. This book is like a fitness manual for the mind. If only they could get their hands on this book, it would change their lives!"

Beau Garraud
Nationally Certified Massage and Bodywork Therapist
Greenville, SC.

"I'm convinced that ADHD shows up in people with genius, as they quickly become bored and frustrated by not having a place to use and develop their intelligence. In this book, Nicky provides key information to refocus that intelligence in such a way to bring peace and satisfaction like never before. I applaud the effort it took to write this book and convey this valuable information. *Train Your Brain* offers hope for anyone suffering from ADHD."

Mitch Jamison
EFT Life Coach, Nationally Certified Massage and Bodywork Therapist
Owner and Director of Back To Basics, Professional Massage Therapy.
www.BTBMassage.com
Tulsa, OK.

"This book is perfect for anyone who wants to conquer their ADHD naturally, without drugs. Nicky shares her personal story of recovery, and offers you hope to do the same with a brain training device called the ALERT. This is a well-organized and well-researched system that provides a viable alternative to drugs. I found this book to be entertaining, easy-to-read and educational. Highly recommended!"

Earma Brown
Author of *Women Of Worth: Become An Extraordinary Woman Using Ordinary Tools, In The Spirit Of Armor Bearing,* and *Write Your Best Book Now.*
www.EarmaBrown.org
Dallas, TX.

"Nicky has experienced an authentic, life-changing transformation with the ALERT brain training program, and you can do the same. I recommend this book for anyone who wants to conquer ADHD."

Lisa Hardwick
Author, *From Broken To Beautiful.*
www.LisaHardwick.com
Urbana-Champaign, IL.

"*Train Your Brain* is informative, innovative, and extremely interesting. This program helps you to focus and organize your brain so you achieve your goals faster and easier."

Lisette Ockeloen
Minneapolis, MN.

"*Train Your Brain* is a must-read for anyone struggling with ADHD. Nicky Vanvalkenburgh pulls back the curtain to reveal how to train your brain and conquer your own unique challenges with ADHD. This should be required reading for every teacher and therapist."

Michelle Matteson
The Maven of The Mind
www.MichelleMatteson.com
www.EasyWayToChange.com
Champaign, IL.

"*Train Your Brain* is very well-written, accurate and informative. I enjoyed the information as well as the conversational tone. This is a very exciting new wave of answers for drugs like Ritalin. Bravo!"

Dr. Caron Goode
Author of *Raising Intuitive Children*.
Winner of National Best Books Awards, Parenting category.
http://www.RaisingIntuitiveChildren.com
http://CoachingParents.wordpress.com
Fort Worth, TX.

"*Train Your Brain* shows you how to overcome stress and regain peace of mind. Plus, it demonstrates how to access peak performance states on demand. I highly recommend this book for anyone who is struggling with ADHD or ADD."

Michael Hutchison
Author of *Megabrain: New Tools And Techniques For Brain Growth And Mind Expansion*; *Megabrain Power*; *The Anatomy Of Sex And Power: An Investigation Of Mind-Body Politics*; *The Book Of Floating: Exploring The Private Sea*, and *Ozone*, Winner of the James Michener & Copernicus Foundation Award.
Santa Fe, NM.

"What I like about Nicky's book is that it's a natural way to train your brain to fit, flexible, and resilient. As a Personal Trainer, coach and radio host, I encourage people to exercise and become more physically fit. I'm excited that Nicky's book does the same thing for the brain."

Laurie Runyan
Certified Personal Trainer, ACE.
Professional Life and Wellness Coach, ICA.
Personal Trainer & Coach, Inner Thinner Peace
Radio Host for Voice America Health & Wellness:
Discovering Your Inner Thinner Peace
www.InnerThinnerPeace.com/
http://www.VoiceAmerica.com/
Avon, IN.

FOREWORD

If you're new to the concept of brain training, it's time to fasten your seat belt. You're about to discover the wild, wacky and wonderful world of audio-visual brain stimulation.

Perhaps I should introduce myself, for those of you who don't know me. My name is Dave Siever. I'm the owner and director of Mind Alive, Inc. in Alberta, Canada. My company manufactures the ALERT brain training device, which is recommended in this book. I designed the ALERT together with school psychologist Michael Joyce in 2000. The device includes special eyeglasses, headphones, and a control box with pre-programmed sessions for ADHD. The ALERT is commonly called a light and sound machine.

Over the years, we've received hundreds of letters, phone calls, and visits from people whose lives are changed by this technology. Students have overcome test anxiety, and went on to make the Dean's List. Business executives have used the technology to sharpen their response time, and think faster on their feet. Lawyers, accountants and stockbrokers have used brain training to relax and de-stress, so they could be more productive at work. Career professionals have used brain training to improve their focus, concentration, and tune out distractions. Housewives and stay-at-home moms have used brain training to supercharge their brainpower, and improve their capacity to think, learn and get things done. Now, it's your turn. You could be the next person to train your brain, and transform your life.

As the title of this book suggests, you can conquer ADHD in 60 days, without Ritalin. There is no need to be dependent upon drugs anymore. With brain training, you can stimulate and arouse your brain naturally, and the results will be longer lasting and more permanent.

There are many forms of brain training on the market today, such as neurofeedback, biofeedback, transcranial magnetic stimulation, cranio-electro stimulation devices, EEG feedback, and neuro-imaging techniques such as quantitative electroencephalography (qEEG). You can also find brain training computer games, brainwave synchronization CDs, and various light and sound machines. All of these things fall under the umbrella of brain training.

What's so special about the ALERT light and sound machine? There are similar devices on the market, but ours has a specific 60-day protocol to help you to conquer ADHD. The ALERT has been sold for several years now, but this is the first book that explains how and why the technology works, so you can determine if it's right for you. Of course, you can also check out Nicky's website at www.TrainYourBrainTransformYourLife.com

My company, Mind Alive, is an electronics manufacturing and design company that incorporated in the province of Alberta, Canada, in 1981. We design and manufacture various audio-visual entrainment (AVE) devices, or light and sound machines. They are used worldwide to assist people from all walks of life to promote better health and increase relaxation.

In addition to ADHD, our devices have proven effective as a non-drug approach to treating chronic pain, fibromyalgia, insomnia, and Pre-Menstrual Syndrome as well as increasing creativity and improving sports and peak-performance. AVE technology has gained popularity because it has been proven to be a quick, safe and effective alternative to many pharmaceutical approaches.

Recently, our AVE devices were licensed by Health Canada as Class I Medical Devices for the treatment of ADHD, Seasonal Affective Disorder (SAD,) depressed mood, insomnia and anxiety. If you live in Canada, you could get a doctor's prescription for our AVE devices, and it may be covered by your health insurance. Mind Alive is the only company that manufactures AVE devices that are licensed by Health Canada. (As of this writing, this arrangement is only available in Canada). Outside of Canada, there is no recognition for AVE devices as a treatment or cure of any medical condition or disability.

We are currently researching the effectiveness of AVE for the treatment of fibromyalgia and chronic pain, insomnia, Attention Deficit Hyperactivity Disorder, Post Traumatic Stress Disorder, and senior's issues such as cognition and frequent falling. Mind Alive continues to research and develop new products. Our products are all thoroughly tested for durability, reliability and effectiveness. Thank you for taking the time to read this book. I'm pleased that you are taking the time to learn more about the ALERT 60-day brain training program for ADHD.

Dave Siever
Owner & Director
Mind Alive, Inc.
www.MindAlive.com
Edmonton, Alberta, Canada.

CONTENTS

CHAPTER SIXTEEN
The Three Rs: Relaxation, Repair And Rejuvenation
Discover how to flip the switch and put the power of relaxation to work

CHAPTER SEVENTEEN
Five Challenges, Five Solutions For ADHD
Here is a final summary of the five things that your brain needs in order

CHAPTERS AT A GLANCE / INTRODUCTION SUMMARIES
"Dear Reader"

APPENDIX

CHAPTER 1

Getting A Jump Start On ADHD

"If modern psychology had existed back then, Thomas Edison would have probably been deemed a victim of ADHD and prescribed a hefty dose of the miracle drug Ritalin. When Edison's mother became aware of his situation, she promptly withdrew him from school and began to home-teach him. Not surprisingly, she was convinced that her son's slightly unusual demeanor and physical appearance were merely outward signs of his remarkable intelligence." —Gerald Beals (1999).

You're about to discover a natural way to conquer Attention Deficit Hyperactivity Disorder (ADHD) in 60 days, without Ritalin. It is a natural remedy that involves training your brain so that you can be more focused, concentrate and remember, get organized, and accomplish more during the day. Some people might say that it sounds too good to be true, but the technology works for me, and it can work for you too.

There are books on the market that teach you how to train your brain with math calculations, memory games, or crossword puzzles. You won't find that approach here! My method of brain training involves lying flat on your back, closing your eyes and using the ALERT light and sound machine for 22 minutes. That's it! This is the lazy way to get rid of ADHD. It's easy, effortless, and effective. The ALERT does all the work for you. If you can spare just 22 minutes a day, then you can train your brain and transform your life. Brain training is a relaxing and enjoyable experience, and it has never been easier to conquer ADHD.

Are you familiar with biofeedback? It's a technique in which you learn to deliberately calm or train your brainwave activity. This book explains a different approach that requires no conscious effort. You won't have to think about it, concentrate, or focus. All you do is close your eyes, relax, and enjoy. You might even zone out or fall asleep. That's okay, because the ALERT light and sound machine is doing all the work.

If you're skeptical, why not read this book first and then decide if this technology is right for you? You see, there is a science behind the technology that makes it work. In the pages to come, you will discover the cause of ADHD— and why it is difficult for you to focus, concentrate, and remember. From the brain's perspective, there is a simple cause for ADHD and a simple solution.

What's the solution for ADHD? To train your brain, of course. ADHD is a sign that your life is out of balance, and you need to fix it. You can fix the imbalance of ADHD by training your brain, and restoring its natural function. If there is nothing wrong with the physical structure of your brain (such as brain damage) then functioning can be restored.

Perhaps your doctor has told you, "There is no cure for ADHD." That simply isn't true. Your doctor may have prescribed Ritalin or another medication. This what it's come down to: You're labeled incurable so it's best that you take pills for the rest of your life? No, this is not your only option! In the pages to come, you will discover how to stimulate and arouse your brain without swallowing pills.

There is a powerhouse tucked under your skull, just waiting to be discovered. Modern science has discovered that the brain is plastic (Doidge, 2007). In other words, your brain has the potential to change or transform itself. The science of brain plasticity enables you to train your brain to think smarter and faster—which is great news for anyone with ADHD.

Inside your brain is everything you need to recover from ADHD. As you train and condition your brain, you will gradually feel a change taking place in your head. Your thoughts will become clearer. It will be easier to focus and concentrate for longer periods of time. You will remember what you've read. Your short term memory will also improve, making it easier to hold onto thoughts that race through your head. In no time, you'll be better organized, more efficient, and more productive. Yes, you have every reason to be upbeat and optimistic about conquering ADHD. It's time to train your brain and transform your life!

Almost everyone knows about Ritalin, but ADHD drugs are not an effective long-term solution. Ritalin is a stimulant drug, but there is another way to stimulate your brain that are equally (if not more) effective. Brain training is a natural, non-invasive way to address the root cause of ADHD, and boost the electro-chemical activity in your brain. Best of all, you'll have fun doing it. You'll actually look forward to your brain training time. It is a relaxing and enjoyable experience, and when you start to get results, the victory will be even sweeter. You'll be so proud of yourself. You'll feel a tremendous sense of pride and accomplishment when you train your brain and transform your life.

Why I Wrote This Book

I wrote this book so that you can discover the technology and understand how and why it works. Brain training has helped thousands of people conquer ADHD. The technology is scientific, powerful, and effective. It should no longer be kept secret. In the pages to come, you will learn about brain training with the ALERT light and sound machine. I will share my personal experience, and explain the science behind the technology. By reading this book, you can examine the facts for yourself and make an informed decision as to whether brain training is right for you.

How I Conquered ADHD,
Lying Flat On My Back, With My Eyes Closed

Finding a natural remedy for ADHD was exciting for me, because I've always struggled with distraction, impulsivity, and not being able to concentrate or focus. When I'm bored, I tend to zone out and disconnect from whatever is happening. A creative imagination can be a good thing, and helps me to think outside the box. Unfortunately, ADHD also causes me to be disorganized, tardy, and lose and forget things. Sometimes, it takes twice as long to get things done.

In college, I was diagnosed with Attention Deficit Disorder (ADD) by a clinical psychologist who ran a battery of tests on me. Being labeled with ADD didn't seem to hold me back— at least, I didn't think so at the time.

By the way, ADD is the old label. The American Psychiatric Association (APA) changed the classification to ADHD, which includes three types of attentional disorders with or without hyperactivity, or the combined type. ADHD is an umbrella term that includes all three types.

Back to my story, I was diagnosed ADD while working on my Master's in counseling and journalism. I made good grades and enjoyed school, but there were a few classes that I wasn't crazy about. For instance, I took a class in Behavioral Statistics that required me to memorize tons of equations and formulas. I was overwhelmed by the long-winded lectures and number-crunching calculations. Sometimes, I could find a way to compensate and make things work. I liked to sit near the front so I could pay attention and be less distracted. I also enjoyed talking to the professor after class. Knowing that I was somebody, not just a number, made all the difference. That little bit of stimulation gave me a boost that I needed to focus and stay on track.

Of course, it wasn't always easy to plug in. When a subject didn't interest me, I tended to daydream or doodle in my notebook. My professor would write equations on the blackboard, and I'd zone out. My eyes glazed over, and I'd start thinking about other things, like lunch or the cute guy sitting nearby. I almost had to slap myself to focus on the material. My brain tended to zone out whenever I wasn't getting enough stimulation. If the class was too difficult, I often felt like giving up. Or, I just wanted to get up and leave. Sometimes, I didn't show up for class at all. When a class didn't interest me, it was difficult to focus on my assignments and get my work done. It's hard to be motivated when I couldn't care less about the subject matter. Before I realized what was happening, I was far behind.

That is why I asked my doctor for a prescription of Ritalin. Some of my friends were already taking it. They mentioned that Ritalin improved their concentration and focus, especially during final exams. I had also heard about Ritalin on TV, newspapers, and in magazines. The media touted Ritalin as a "smart drug" or "cognitive enhancer." It seemed pretty harmless, so why not try it? To my surprise, the medicine worked like a charm. I found myself reading at turbo speed and whipping through my statistics assignments. Feelings of overwhelm and frustration melted away. No more procrastination or feeling unmotivated! I almost felt like the Bionic Woman with super powers. I could study, memorize, and write at an accelerated rate. Nothing could stop me.

Yes, I was flying high with Ritalin. But when the medicine wore off, I came crashing down fast. Tears streamed down my face and I felt incredibly sad. All my energy had been drained away. Why me and why now? I still had homework to do, reading assignments, and papers to write. Of course, I could take another pill. That would get me up again, but then I was so wired that I couldn't sleep. There were other side effects: Stomachaches, acne, constipation, and dry mouth— but the worst part was the jitters and sadness that accompanied the Ritalin tapering off.

Another side effect was that my mind got stuck in a continuous loop. Have you ever dreamed about the same thing over and over? Or perhaps you have a CD that is scratched up or damaged. When you play the CD, it skips. The music gets stuck at a certain place. The same section repeats itself. This is what often happened to me when Ritalin wore off. It was a strange withdrawal or rebound experience. I found myself obsessing about stupid things. For instance, I'd re-check my school assignments that I already completed. Did I really complete the work, or were parts of it unfinished?

As a psychology major, I recognized my symptoms were obsessive compulsive. There was a girl in my class who was like that. She took five showers a day, and constantly washed her hands. I remember her telling me, "I just can't get clean. I scrub and wash myself, but I still feel dirty afterwards."

I didn't have that problem, but my looping tendency was getting out of hand. At night, my dreams were also stuck in a loop. I'd tell myself, "Snap out it! Enough already!" But the dreams wouldn't stop, like a bad movie that repeats itself.

I hated Ritalin, and what it was doing to me. The side effects were getting more and more bizarre. Something inside me screamed, "No more Ritalin! It's just not worth it!" My life was becoming a roller coaster and I wanted to get off. There had to be a better way.

I was also fed-up with doctor's visits, running to the pharmacy for refills, and shelling out the co-payments. It was time-consuming and expensive. Plus, I wasn't getting any better. I was sedated, but not cured. The medicine took care of my ADHD symptoms, but when it wore off I was back at square one. Nothing had changed!

I tried other ADHD medications such as Adderall and Dexadrine, but my response was exactly the same. I loved the positive effects, but coming down from the meds was like taking a nosedive, looping upside down and going backwards in the dark. It wasn't a fun ride anymore; it was scary. I decided to step on the brakes and stop the meds entirely.

I read everything about ADD and ADHD that I could find, including books on neuroscience and brain power. I switched to brain vitamins and herbs, which improved my energy levels, but I always craved an extra push.

Ultimately, I earned my Master's, graduated with honors, and began working full-time. Fifteen years later, I discovered something that changed my life forever. My friend Morry told me about the ALERT light and sound machine. "I'm coming out of that ADHD fog, and seeing the light at the end of the tunnel," he said.

"I'm getting the positive effects of Ritalin, without swallowing pills. I can read better, concentrate and focus, listen to public speakers, and remember it all!" he said.

Morry explained that the ALERT was a home-based brain training program for ADHD. It consists of headphones, funky eyeglasses, and a control box with pre-programmed sessions. I'll never forget what Morry said, "You can train your brain to conquer ADHD, and it's so easy that you can do it lying flat on your back, with your eyes closed!"

Intrigued, I purchased an ALERT for myself. I was skeptical, but figured it was worth a try. If this device could help me get a grip on my ADHD, then it would be worth every penny.

Using the ALERT wasn't anything like I expected it to be. I closed my eyes and noticed the mild flashing lights and heartbeat sounds. It seemed odd, but the rhythm was gentle and soothing. I felt relaxed and at ease. My mind chatter, or internal dialogue, seemed to slow down and become quiet. My thoughts faded to black, and I fell asleep. The session was over 22 minutes later.

Upon waking, I looked at the clock on my nightstand. I felt well-rested, as if I'd slept all night. Funny thing, it was the middle of the day, and I'd only taken a short nap. I felt warm, cozy, and relaxed. There was a yellow coffee mug on my nightstand, and it looked very three-dimensional, almost like a beautiful painting. I got up and looked out the window. To my surprise, the neighbors' houses looked different. It was as if I'd stepped into a pop-up storybook. The houses looked more three-dimensional. It was as if someone had tied a string to the houses and pulled them up. I'd never noticed the houses looking like that before. I didn't understand what was happening to me, but it was something good. I felt euphoric, but also calm and focused.

I remember thinking, "Hmm, maybe I could put this energy to good use." I went to my desk and reviewed my to-do list. I quickly got busy with my assignments and finished a book that I was reading. Amazingly, I wasn't distracted or preoccupied. Instead, I had energy and stamina, as if I was in a state of flow. It was amazing how productive I was after using the ALERT.

I continued to use the ALERT every day, for the next two months. Sometimes I'd use the ALERT after exercising at the gym. I attend group fitness classes, which are often intense cardio workouts. Afterwards, my clothes are soaking wet and I feel exhausted, but I always have work waiting for me on my desk. I also run an internet business out of my home, which keeps me busy. Using the ALERT gives me a 22-minute power nap. It helps me to relax deeply, and awake refreshed and ready to focus on my work.

The ALERT is also handy for stress relief. It is easy to get overwhelmed by deadlines and responsibilities. Feeling overwhelmed makes it hard to think straight and be productive. Under pressure, I tend to make careless mistakes. The ALERT gives me a 22-minute stress reduction session. As I relax deeply, I let go of my worries and frustration. My mind chatter slows down and becomes quiet. This relaxation response takes the edge off of stress. It enables me to tap into my creative muse, rather than my inner critic.

The ALERT is a quick and easy way to get a grip on my ADHD. I use the device in the comfort of my own home, which is convenient and hassle-free. The benefits include energizing my brain to read, study or solve problems; boosting my mood, helping me to calm down, relax and stabilize my emotions; and to help reduce stress and anxiety. All of these things enable me to be more productive with my work.

Now that I've completed the ALERT 60-day program, I can honestly say that it's made a tremendous difference in my life. Morry was right. Brain training with the ALERT was so easy that I could do it with my eyes closed. There were no side effects and I'll never ride the Ritalin roller coaster again. The ALERT helped me to conquer my ADHD and you can discover it too.

The Science Behind The Technology

You might be wondering if my recovery from ADHD is the result of the placebo effect, power of suggestion, or just getting lucky. Actually, there is a science behind the technology. The ALERT light and sound machine has a specifically designed protocol for ADHD that is safe, reliable, and effective. As you read this book, you will discover how and why the technology works. Very briefly, the ALERT addresses five things that your brain needs in order to overcome ADHD:

1. **Your brain needs to improve it's electro-chemical communication.** ADHD is a wiring and firing problem. By improving the electro-chemical communication in your brain, you will think clearer, faster, and smarter. *Fixing this shortcoming will be so easy that you can do it with your eyes closed!*

2. **Your brainwaves need to get up-to-speed.** Either your brainwaves are sluggish (too slow), hyperactive (too fast), or somewhere in between. The trick is correcting this imbalance, so the speed of your brainwaves is within a normal range. *By the time you finish reading this book, you'll know how to get the tempo exactly right.*

3. **Your brain needs to learn the Rhythm of Peak Performance.** Having ADHD is like being rhythmically challenged. You're out of step with the rhythm of focusing, concentrating, and remembering information. *You'll be amazed at what happens when you get in-synch with the Rhythm of Peak Performance.*

4. Your brain needs stimulation, conditioning, and exercise.
Researchers have found that people with ADHD tend to have "low arousal," or "sleepy" brains. That's why it's pure torture to listen to a boring lecture or wait in line. Boring activities don't challenge, stimulate, or arouse your brain. *By reading this book, you'll discover how to get the stimulation that your brain craves.*

5. Your brain needs the three Rs: Relaxation, restoration and rejuvenation. If you're bogged down by stress, your brain will work less, which is when you need it the most. *If you feel overwhelmed, just close your eyes and "chill-lax" that stress right out of your head. This book will show you how.*

In the pages to come, I will explain more about these five brain boosters. They may seem strange now, but by the time you finish reading this book, these concepts will be crystal-clear. With the help of these five brain boosters, you can train your brain and transform your life.

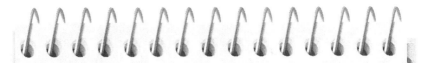

Dear Reader,

Do you feel overwhelmed? You might be looking at this book and wondering if these pages will hold your interest. Adults with ADHD often report difficulty in maintaining their focus long enough to read an entire book. If this is true for you, don't worry. You shouldn't feel obligated to read from cover to cover. Depending on your circumstances, you may not choose to read every chapter.

To gauge your interest, you can read these letters. At the start of each chapter, I'll give you a quick summary, and then you can decide whether to continue reading or move on to a topic that is more relevant for you.

The next chapter covers ten warning signs of ADHD:

1. Poor concentration
2. Distraction
3. Disorganization
4. Restlessness
5. Low arousal
6. Craving for stimulation
7. Impulsiveness
8. Poor short-term memory
9. Dissatisfaction and frustration
10. Emotionally wounded

(Continued)

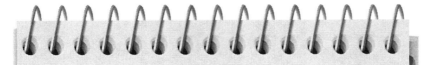

Do these "warning signs" sound familiar? If so, then you probably have ADHD.

What you're experiencing is not imaginary. ADHD is a real problem, but there is also a real solution for it. There is no need to be overwhelmed, confused, or frustrated any longer.

In this book, I will give you specific techniques and strategies to help you train your brain and transform your life. I know some of you are thinking, "That's impossible!" but I assure you it isn't. Thousands of people have successfully used the ALERT brain training program to conquer their ADHD and so can you.

My friend, the days of being held back by ADHD are over. This time, it's going to be different. You're going to break the rules and do things your way. No more drugs and doctors in white coats. No more roller coaster rides. No more suffering either. You'll be doing things the easy way— in less time, with less effort. It's time to train your brain and transform your life!

All the best,
Nicky

CHAPTER 2

ADHD & The DSM-IV

"When the notion of retraining the brain was first discussed, traditional physicians bristled: 'You can't train the brain; we need a medication to speed it up or slow it down.' Almost everything in medicine ultimately boils down to cutting something out or giving a pill— The cut-and-poison track. In contrast to this, there is a wonderful concept in complementary medicine: Human potential. What are human beings ultimately capable of? Why can't humans learn to cure themselves by learning to unlock the secret of what is going on inside the body?"
—Robert W. Hill & Eduardo Castro (2002), *Getting Rid Of Ritalin.*

ADHD has many faces— from the student who is struggling to pass a boring class, to the stay-at-home Mom who feels "all-over-the-place" and can't seem to get organized, to the employee who can't seem to finish a project that he's been working on for months. If you know or suspect that you have ADHD or ADD, then I want to help you get past your pain, confusion, and anxiety.

In this book, I will give you specific techniques and strategies to help you train your brain and transform your life. I know some of you are thinking, "That's impossible," but I assure you it isn't. Thousands of people have successfully used the ALERT brain training program to conquer their ADHD and so can you.

If you have ADHD, you've probably taken Ritalin or another stimulant medicine. We'll talk more about medication later on, but I imagine that you're fed up and want a real solution. You want something that is effective and long lasting. Something that won't wear off and take you back to square one. Something that you can build upon and maintain for a lifetime. Something that takes you to the next level and transforms you into the person that you really want to be.

You're tired of being a lowly caterpillar, crawling on your belly and inhaling dust. That is why you're wrapping yourself up in a cocoon. As you close your eyes and rest, a metamorphosis is taking place. Soon, you will emerge as a beautiful butterfly. You will spread your wings and fly. A new adventure awaits. As you soar through the air, you realize that every second that you spent waiting for your transformation has been worthwhile. Finally, you are free to be everything that you've always dreamed of being.

Yes, the days of being held back by ADHD are over. This time, it's going to be different. You're going to break the rules and do things your way. No more drugs and doctors in white coats. No more roller coaster rides. No more suffering either. You'll be doing things the easy way— in less time, with less effort.

You'll be getting rid of your ADHD, while lying flat on your back, with your eyes closed. It takes just 22 minutes. You'll probably drift off off and wake up when it's over. You'll know exactly what you're doing, and that you're still in control. Actually, you'll be on your way to a life without ADHD. You'll be sitting behind the wheel, on your way to a new destination— a place far, far away— where ADHD is nothing but a distant memory. This magical place is real, and it's not for someday, woulda, coulda, shoulda, or "Why didn't I?" It's for right now. You're in the right place, at the right time, and this program is for you.

My friend, you're on your way to becoming the person you've always wanted to be. After 60 days with the ALERT brain training program, you will have some pep in your step. Your thoughts will become clearer. It will be easier to focus and concentrate for longer periods of time. You will remember what you've read. Your short-term memory will also improve, making it easier to hold on to thoughts that race through your head. In no time, you'll be better organized, more efficient, and more productive. Plus, you'll have more energy than you ever imagined.

Before we can get to the solution, we need to define the problem. Here is a short list of ADHD symptoms, loosely adapted from the American Psychiatric Association's *Diagnostic and Statistics Manual*, or DSM-IV (2010).

Ten Warning Signs Of Attention Deficit Hyperactivity Disorder

1. **Poor concentration.** You're like a light switch. You're turned off whenever something is boring, too complicated, or hard to understand. You just don't have enough of a boost to focus and stay on track. Unless something interests you, it's hard to concentrate and focus. Over-focus can also be a problem, causing you to dwell on things (rather than letting go and moving on).

2. **Distraction.** You're easily distracted. If something doesn't capture your attention, then you tune out. You start thinking about other things. Part of the problem is a lack of stimulation. If you don't have enough stimulation (or arousal) then your thoughts will be elsewhere.

3. **Disorganization.** You tend to be all-over-the-place and scattered. Your workspace is messy. Perhaps you're a pack rat who doesn't like to get rid of anything. You lose or misplace things. Getting organized is a big chore, and it's hard for you to come up with a game plan for getting things done. Sometimes, you put things off because you feel overwhelmed. Creative ideas come to you quickly, but putting the pieces together is a challenge. You can't figure out how to get things done in a fast, efficient, and organized way. Sometimes, it's easier to quit then to keep going. You hate being disorganized, and feel stuck in a rut. You aren't sure how to make things better, either. Another challenge is time management: Being on-time, doing too many things at once, and underestimating how long it takes to complete a task.

4. **Restlessness.** You have a low tolerance for boredom. Waiting in line is pure torture. If you're listening to a boring speaker, you'd like to get up and leave. You prefer sound bites to long-winded explanations. By the way, why do some people take so long to get to the point? They're driving you crazy. Part of the problem is that you have nervous energy. Sometimes, your mind chatters or races, distracting you from getting things done. Restlessness is also evident when you can't sit still, or you're tapping your fingers or feet. If you have a lot of your mind, you're likely to be wound up, wired and wide awake.

5. **Low arousal.** You can't seem to get into gear. You're bored or feel apathetic. For some reason, you have trouble starting projects, switching

between activities, or finishing your work. If something doesn't interest or challenge you, then you might as well forget it.

6. **Craving for stimulation.** Perhaps you're a thrill seeker or adrenaline junkie. This gives you an extra push that helps you to focus. You crave stimulation and there's nothing like a little excitement to stir things up. You look for ways to turn on your brain power. You might drink coffee, soda, or energy drinks. Whatever it takes, you need a boost to get yourself up and ready for action. You might even pick a fight, run around the room, scream at the top of your lungs, or do something else to get yourself into gear. Sometimes, a little excitement is just what you need to turn on your brainpower.

7. **Impulsiveness.** You blurt out whatever comes to mind, without thinking first. Sometimes, you do or say things that you later regret. You might butt in on other people's conversations. Your impulsiveness may also be evident when you're driving. You may drive too fast, run stop signs or red lights, or get angry with other drivers. At work, you might quit or give up because of minor conflicts or frustration. In personal relationships, you might end things suddenly or make impulsive commitments. Sometimes, impulsiveness makes reading difficult. You give up easily, because the material is complicated, hard to understand, or doesn't get to the point immediately.

8. **Poor short-term memory**. You have good insights—but sometimes, your thoughts race by so fast that you can't make sense of them. You enter into a room to get something, and then immediately forget what it was. You lose track because you can't seem to hold on to your thoughts long enough. This is a short-term memory problem. Another problem is reading something and then immediately forgetting what you've just read. It's like not having enough RAM (Random Access Memory) in your computer. If you don't have enough RAM, your computer may be slow, give you error messages, or shut down. The same thing happens with your brain when you have a poor short-term memory. Your brain doesn't seem to be operating at peak capacity.

9. **Dissatisfaction and frustration**. You might to be performing below your ability. Or perhaps you're employed below your ability. You do a mediocre job when you're capable of much more. It all adds up to

frustration and disillusionment with life. You'd like to accomplish more, but you're not sure how to make things happen. It's frustrating when there is a huge gap between where you are and where you want to be.

10. **Emotionally wounded.** The harder you try, the worse things get. You feel like giving up. ADHD is emotionally draining and overwhelming. Sometimes you hate yourself and wonder if things will ever get better. How can you be optimistic about the future when ADHD keeps holding you back from being all that you can be?

If you recognize at least six of these symptoms, then you probably have ADHD. What you're experiencing is not imaginary. ADHD is a real problem, but there is also a real solution for it. There is no need to be overwhelmed, confused, or frustrated any longer. This book will show you how to train your brain and transform your life, so that you can conquer ADHD in 60 days, without Ritalin.

For the purposes of this book, ADHD is defined as these ten symptoms. This is my working definition of ADHD. Yes, it's slightly different from the official DSM-IV classification. Their main classification is ADHD with three subtypes: "Predominately Inattentive" (usually called ADD), "Predominately Hyperactive-Impulsive," and the "Combined Type."

As I mentioned before, the DSM-IV uses ADHD as an umbrella term to cover all three subtypes. Whenever the term ADHD is used, it includes ADD, Predominately Hyperactive-Impulsive, and the Combined Type.

My definition of ADHD is different in that it clusters the symptoms into one list. When it comes to using the ALERT, it does not matter if you're hyperactive or not. The ALERT brain training program will benefit any-one who wants less ADHD (or ADD) and more brainpower. If you want to train your brain for peak performance, then the ALERT is for you.

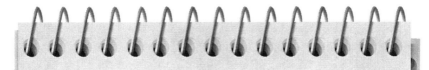

Dear Reader,

The topic of ADHD is confusing! There are various opinions and points of view. Consider the differences between medical doctors, psychologists, psychiatrists, neurotherapists, and biofeedback practitioners. Each of them diagnose and treat ADHD differently. It's a hot topic, with authorities on opposite sides of the fence.

It's important to think for ourselves, and do our own homework. Don't fall into a trap of blindly trusting authorities. This is the mistake that I made when taking Ritalin. I assumed the drug was safe and mild. I assumed my doctor had my best interests at heart. Now I realize that my doctor only has a partial understanding. He doesn't know everything. It's a hard lesson to learn. Just because someone is an authority does not mean they're right. Sometimes, an authority isn't correct at all.

If you've been diagnosed with ADHD, there are certain assumptions that go hand-in-hand with that label. Unfortunately, many of these assumptions are wrong! I'm convinced that ADHD:

- Isn't a neurological disease.
- Isn't a sign that you're defective.
- Isn't a devastating life sentence.

(Continued)

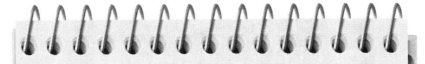

Plus, ADHD does not equal:

- A medical need for Ritalin.
- A dependency on drugs.

When it comes to brain training, you might be hesitant to try it because you want scientific evidence and proof that it works. That's why I wrote this book: To share the science, mixed with personal stories, insights, and experiences. It's satisfying and comforting to have scientific support for brain training, but most people simply want to feel better. Deep down inside, that's all we really want. We want to feel better. We also want compassion and understanding, not just a bunch of information. When it comes down to it, that's what really matters.

There will always be critics who frown upon brain training, and insist that drugs are the only way to go. Ultimately, it doesn't matter what the critics say. The ALERT is a clinically-tested method that is safe, reliable, easy, and effective. It fits the medical credo of "First, do no harm." There are no known side effects. Of course, it's not the only drug-free approach to ADHD. But it's worked for me, and it can work for you too.

All the best,
Nicky

CHAPTER 3

ADHD & "The Elephant And Six Blind Men"

Once upon a time, there lived six blind men in a village. One day, the villagers told them, "Hey, there is an elephant in the village today."

They had no idea what an elephant was. They decided, "Even though we would not be able to see it, let us go and feel it anyway." All of them went where the elephant was. Every one of them touched the elephant.

"Hey, the elephant is a pillar," said the first man, who touched the leg of the elephant.

"Oh, no! It's like a rope," said the second man, who touched the tail.

"No, it's like a thick branch of a tree," said the third man, who touched the trunk of the elephant.

"It's like a big fan that you'd use to keep yourself cool," said the fourth man, who touched the ear of the elephant.

"It's like a huge wall," said the fifth man, who touched the belly of the elephant.

"No, it's like a solid pipe," said the sixth man, who touched the tusk of the elephant.

They began to argue about the elephant, and each one of them insisted that he was right. They were all getting agitated. A wise man was passing by and he saw this. He stopped and asked them, "What's the matter?"

They said, "We cannot agree on what the elephant is like." Each one of them told what he thought the elephant resembled. The wise man calmly explained to them, "All of you are right. The reason every one of you is telling it differently is because each one of you touched a different part of the elephant. So, actually the elephant has all those features that you described."

"Oh!" everyone said. There was no more fighting. They felt happy that they were all partly right (Jainism Global Resource Center, 2010).

"The Elephant And The Blind Men" is a simple but profound story. Each one of the men touched a different part of the elephant, and came to a different conclusion. Each man was firmly convinced that he alone was correct. However, each man was only partly right.

The story suggests that people see things in different ways, based on their experience and perspective. No one knows everything there is to know about a particular subject. Even an expert may not be aware of the whole picture. What we know is imperfect and incomplete. "We see through a glass darkly," suggests the Bible (1 Corinthians 13:12).

"The Elephant And The Blind Men" could also be applied to ADHD. Consider the differences between medical doctors, psychologists, psychiatrists, neurotherapists, and biofeedback practitioners. Obviously, these experts are not physically blind, but they do diagnose and treat ADHD differently.

Psychologists diagnose ADHD based on a battery of tests, such as the Quick Test, Test of Variables of Attention (TOVA), Integrated Visual and Auditory Continuous Performance Test (IVA), and Conners' Continuous Performance Test. A psychologist diagnoses you based on your answers to questions, marked checklists, and performance on computer-based tests. Unfortunately, it is easy to skew, manipulate, or distort your responses. "Yes, I'm distracted most of the time," you might admit. The psychologist marks your responses. If you have a lot of ADHD symptoms, then you're diagnosed with ADHD. Treatment includes psychological counseling and making a doctor's appointment to obtain ADHD medication.

Medical doctors diagnose ADHD based on what their patients tell them. Sometimes doctors insist that their patients be professionally tested for ADHD, in order to document the diagnosis for insurance claims. Sometimes, they do a medical exam to rule out other causes. Typically, doctors prescribe drugs for ADHD. When it comes to children, most doctors spend less than an hour making an evaluation before prescribing Ritalin (Wingert, 1996).

Psychiatrists diagnose ADHD based on symptoms and medical history. They may use a battery of tests. Ultimately, diagnosis is made on the basis of the DSM-IV definition of ADHD. Of course, a psychiatrist is a medical doctor who has also received advanced training in psychology. Psychiatrists usually prescribe drugs for ADHD.

Meanwhile, a growing number of professionals are looking at ADHD from the brain's perspective. Psychiatrist Daniel Amen (2002) makes a compelling case for the existence of ADHD using a nuclear medicine technique called "Single Photon Emission Computed Tomography" or SPECT. Dr. Amen uses SPECT to scan people's brains and objectively test for ADHD. From more than 8,000 such studies and more than 12,000 patient evaluations, Dr. Amen concludes that six different types of ADHD exist.

Biofeedback diagnoses and treats ADHD based on body signals. It involves hooking you up to equipment that measures your heart rate (which rises with arousal) or skin conductance (the more you sweat, the easier it is to pass a mild current through your body).

Treatment for ADHD involves learning to relax using a biofeedback machine. The biofeedback machine might be an advanced computer game, or a computer monitor with simple images, such as bar graphs. Either way, the computer screen lets you know whether your arousal is increasing or decreasing. The goal is learning to relax using feedback from the machine.

Neurofeedback is a variation on biofeedback. Neurofeedback diagnoses and treats ADHD based on the measurement of brainwaves. Your brainwaves change with whatever you're doing. The presence of different brainwave frequencies indicates whether you are concentrating or distracted.

Neurotherapists use a "quantitative electroencephalogram" (qEEG) to measure the electrical activity of the brain. It's a painless, non-invasive procedure that involves placing small electrodes on your head. The electrodes read the tiny voltages (brainwaves) produced by brain activity. These signals are amplified, digitally analyzed, and interpreted on the computer screen as colored-coded brain maps. These brain maps provide information about brainwave activity. Your information is then fed into a database to determine how you compare to a normal functioning brain. The computer analysis provides information about all of the brainwave bands: Delta, theta, beta and alpha (Hill & Castro, 2002).

Usually, neurofeedback for ADHD involves going to a special clinic one or two times per week. The patient is connected to a specialized EEG computer with a monitor, and plays a computer game. The game teaches you to speed up or slow down your brainwave patterns. It does this by rewarding healthy brainwave activity. The game uses "operant conditioning techniques" to teach you how to speed up your brainwaves. Brain imaging techniques are used to assess your ADHD before and after treatment. Also available are home-based neurofeedback games, which are played on the computer.

Do I Need To Be Professionally Tested For ADHD?

There are a variety of ways to test for ADHD: Psychological tests, brain scans, body signals, and brainwaves. It makes you wonder, "Do I need to be professionally tested for ADHD? Or is it enough to look at the list of symptoms, and determine whether or not I have ADHD?"

Actually, the diagnosis of ADHD is very subjective. There is no official blood, saliva, or urine test for ADHD. Perhaps a lab test or physical exam would make the diagnosis more objective and scientific. Consider what Dr. Mary Ann Block (2001), a physician from Texas, says in her book, *No More ADHD*:

"When I was a guest on the Montel Williams Show, there was also a psychiatrist on the show. The psychiatrist was supporting the use of drugs for ADHD and I was discussing the fact that there are many underlying health problems that can cause the same symptoms. On the show, I mentioned that I rarely see a child who has had a physical exam, much less lab work, before being diagnosed with ADHD and prescribed mind-altering drugs. And then, on national television, the psychiatrist said, "Look, we're psychiatrists. It's a psychiatric diagnosis. Psychiatric diagnoses are based on the history. Psychiatrists don't do physical exams."

"I know from experience that many doctors don't do physicals exams before prescribing psychiatric drugs, so I was glad that this psychiatrist shared this with all who were watching that day. My clinical experience confirms that this is usually what occurs to children who are diagnosed with ADHD. They see a doctor, but the doctor does not do a physical exam or look for any health or learning problems before giving the child an ADHD diagnosis and a prescription drug. This is not how I was taught to practice medicine. In my medical education, I was taught to do a complete history and physical exam. I was taught to consider something called a differential diagnosis. To do this, one must consider all possible underlying causes of the symptoms" (Block, 2001, p. 10).

Evidently, most people are diagnosed with ADHD based on personal observations. Doctors may diagnose you as having ADHD without a physical exam or psychological tests. Instead, they make an assessment based on the criteria of the DSM-IV.

Dr. Block (2010) also claims that ADHD is a made-up diagnosis:

"No one found it under a microscope. No one discovered it from a lab test. It doesn't show up in urine or blood. You can't find it anywhere in the body. You're not going to believe this, but it's true! A group of psychiatrists get together every few years at their national convention and sit down in a room and decide what behaviors they think should be considered psychiatric disorders. Then this group of psychiatrists vote to include certain groups of behaviors as psychiatric disorders and make up names for these disorders. Then they include this new disorder in the next edition of the DSM, a Billing Bible for insurance companies, which lists psychiatric disorders and the symptoms used to describe them.

"Are you shocked? I was when I learned about it. Psychiatrists write a book and decide what behaviors or groups of behaviors will go in their book and then they give them a name, like Attention Deficit Hyperactivity Disorder. Once this is done, they have a new disorder, a code number to bill insurance companies for it, and psychiatric drugs to treat it. Every child that has these behaviors is then at risk of being labeled with ADHD.

"That's exactly what happened. Within one year of deciding to insert ADHD in the DSM, 500,000 children in the United States were diagnosed with the disorder and today the number is closer to five million. Through a simple vote, with no objective means to define this psychiatric label, a new disorder is born and begins to take on a life of its own. There is no objective way to define or to diagnose these made-up diagnoses. If you have high blood pressure, your doctor can objectively measure and diagnose the problem. If you have diabetes, your doctor can objectively measure your blood sugar and give you a diagnosis. There is no way to measure for a psychiatric diagnosis" (Block, 2010).

Confused? Me too. After digging through the literature, I discovered Dr. Block is correct. The APA voted ADD in as a "mental disorder" by a show of hands (majority vote) in 1980 at their committee meeting, without scientific evidence present. It was placed in the DSM-III (Third Edition). Later, they changed the label to ADHD. In 1987, ADHD was voted in by a similar show of hands (majority vote) as well and placed into the DSM-IV (Fourth Edition). Neither of these committee meetings presented scientific evidence that ADHD is the result of brain malfunction, disease, chemical imbalance, neurobiological conditions, or illness. Yet, all of these are popular ways that ADHD is coined and marketed today (ADHD Testing, 2010).

Even the National Institutes of Health admits that, "We do not have an independent, valid test for ADHD, and there is no data to indicate that ADHD is due to a brain malfunction" (Herring, 2010).

When it comes down to it, ADHD is a very confusing diagnosis. Even experts disagree. Every one of the aforementioned disciplines (medicine, psychiatry, psychology, biofeedback, and neurotherapy) is different. Each discipline establishes its own parameters, and works within these parameters. These parameters help experts to test and validate their hypothesis. That's good, but the disadvantage is that it is easy to become blind to other parameters.

By the way, there is nothing wrong with questioning the validity of an authority. Far too often, we blindly trust authorities. We trust what they say because they have a title or advanced expertise. We assume they're smarter than we are. After all, they're well-educated and have impressive credentials. They've spent time doing research and documenting the issues. Surely, they know what is right and best.

In reality, authorities make wrong assumptions and wrong conclusions. An authority may only have a partial understanding (like the blind men who touched the elephant). Sometimes, an authority isn't correct at all. Just because someone is an authority does not mean they're right.

Personally, I fell into this trap when I took Ritalin. I accepted the ADD diagnosis and drug treatment without question. I never questioned the psychologist or doctor. Looking back, I now realize that I was like a sheep going down a gated chute to be slaughtered. I never challenged the authorities. I didn't do my own research, or ask tough questions. Like millions of people, I took Ritalin because everyone else was doing it.

Whatever Tool You Use Determines The Diagnosis

Psychologist Abraham Maslow once said, "If all you have is a hammer, everything looks like a nail" (Law of the Instrument, 2010).

In the same way, an authority's tool of choice influences the way they define, diagnose and treat ADHD. A psychologist's tools are the DSM-IV, psychological tests and counseling. The tools of medical doctors and psychiatrists are the DSM-IV, symptoms, and medical history. Both of these approaches look at a person's behavior to diagnose ADHD, and treatment usually involves drugs.

Meanwhile, biofeedback and neurofeedback practitioners also use the DSM-IV to define ADHD, but they have expanded their arsenal of tools by taking a closer look at the brain.

Biofeedback claims that certain body signals are typical of ADHD. Neurofeedback suggests that certain brainwave frequencies and brainwave patterns are indications of ADHD. Both biofeedback and neurofeedback use this information (body signals or brainwaves) to tackle ADHD, in lieu of drug treatment. Meanwhile, Dr. Mary Ann Block has a different set of tools, and offers a different treatment. She also offers a drug-free way to address ADHD.

Different Tools, Different Approach

Each expert has a different set of tools, and takes a different approach. And what about people who figure it out on their own? You may read the DSM-IV definition of ADHD, and diagnose yourself: "Hmm, I'm easily distracted, disorganized, have trouble focusing and concentrating, and I have plenty of restless energy. Ok, now I understand why. It's because I have ADHD or ADD."

Whether you're self-diagnosed or professionally diagnosed, one thing is certain. We understand parts of the elephant, but there is much more to the animal than what we see, feel and experience. Everyone's understanding is partial. We may understand parts of ADHD, but no one knows everything.

What's Wrong With Labeling Someone ADHD Or ADD?

There is nothing wrong with the DSM-IV definition of ADHD, but some people are quick to jump to conclusions. There are at least six false assumptions that often go hand-in-hand with the ADHD label. Let's review these assumptions, so that we can take a fresh look at what ADHD is (and what it isn't).

(1) **ADHD isn't a neurological disease.** Don't believe anyone who tells you that ADHD is a disease like cancer or diabetes. That's a lie, a falsehood, and an invalid assumption. ADHD is nothing more than a list of symptoms. If you have ADHD, you are not mentally ill. You're simply a person who is distractible, restless, impulsive, and struggles to concentrate.

(2) **ADHD does not equal a medical need for Ritalin.** You may encounter this line of reasoning: "If your child needed eyeglasses, you wouldn't think twice about getting them." Or, "If you have diabetes, I bet you'd take insulin. It's the same thing with ADHD, so why think twice about taking Ritalin?"

The not-so-subtle implication is that you're being negligent if you don't medicate your ADHD child. Likewise, adults with ADHD are irresponsible if they don't take their medicine. In reality, ADHD isn't a disease, and it doesn't require drug treatment.

(3) **ADHD drugs are not safe.** Most people assume that Ritalin is safe and mild, because it is often prescribed for children. In reality, Ritalin is an amphetamine that is pharmacologically similar to cocaine. It's addictive and causes severe withdrawal symptoms and side effects.

(4) **ADHD is not a sign that you're defective.** Ritalin/ADHD advocates claim that your brain is like a sports car with defective brakes (Quinn & Stern, 1991). They say you need Ritalin to control yourself. Without Ritalin, you're driving a car without brakes, and are headed for disaster. Sadly, the implication is that you're out-of-control, and are powerless to do anything but swallow pills.

This book takes a different approach. Think of your brain as a car that needs a jump start. Brain training is like hooking up the black and red jumper cables on your car battery, and getting recharged. Instead of drugs, you're using your brain's natural electricity to ramp up (and energize) your brain for peak performance. With ADHD, you're not defective— you just need a jump start.

(5) **ADHD is not a devastating life sentence.** Being diagnosed with a psychiatric label implies there is something seriously wrong with you. To make matters worse, you're told there is nothing you can do about it. When making these assumptions, it's common sense that you (1) accept your disability, (2) learn to live with it, (3) stay on your meds to keep the situation under control.

This line of reasoning suggests, "There's no cure for ADHD. The best thing you can do is take Ritalin for the rest of your life." Wrong, wrong, wrong! In reality, you can train your brain and transform your life. You're not a victim of ADHD. You can be victorious over it.

(6) **ADHD shouldn't create a dependency on drugs.** When you go back to your doctor for refills, you're dependent upon your doctor. You're dependent upon your pharmacist. You're dependent upon the pills. You've got to keep coming back for more. It's a dependency that costs you time, energy and money. Plus, you've lost control. You're no longer in

control of your brain and behavior— the drugs are doing it for you. It's time to take your power back. That is why I've written this book. I want you to conquer ADHD in 60 days, without Ritalin. In the pages to come, I'll share with you the difference it's made in my life. Brain training with the ALERT light and sound machine has enabled me to be less distracted, better organized, and more productive. It has transformed my life, and can do the same for you.

The ALERT fits the medical credo of "First, do no harm." Brain training is a harmless tool that has no known side effects. Of course, it's not the only drug-free approach to ADHD. But it's worked for me, and it's proven to be effective for thousands of other people. It's a method of brain training that is rooted in neurotherapy, and is backed up with an impressive review of literature. It is a clinically-tested method that is safe, reliable, easy, and effective.

By the way, I don't claim to know all the answers. There are plenty of valid ways to cope with ADHD that are not covered in this book. I've tried to limit the scope of this book to the elephant of ADHD, and the brain training program that has helped me to conquer my symptoms.

Sometimes people are hesitant to try new things, because they want scientific evidence and proof that it works. That's why I wrote this book: To share the science, mixed with personal stories, insights and experiences. It's satisfying and comforting to have scientific support for brain training, but most people simply want to feel better. Deep down inside, that's all we really want. We want to feel better. We also want compassion and understanding, not just a bunch of information.

My critics might say that I'm a blind lady who is only looking at one part of the elephant, but that doesn't matter. What matters is that I've found something that dramatically reduces my ADHD symptoms, and has changed my life for the better. What matters is that you can do the same. You can tackle those stubborn ADHD symptoms, like distraction, disorganization, restless energy, and low arousal. You can tackle these symptoms without swallowing pills or wrestling with side effects. My friend, if you can spare just 22 minutes a day, then you can train your brain and transform your life. Yes, you can conquer ADHD in 60 days, without Ritalin. When it comes down to it, that's what really matters.

Dear Reader,

The next chapter shows you how to get up and running with the ALERT brain training system. The goal is to do one 22-minute session a day. Do a session for five days, and then go on to the next session. To keep track of your progress, use the chart in the back of this book.

Biofeedback practitioner Anna Wise (2002) claims there are six stages that occur during deep relaxation. As you use the ALERT, you'll gradually progress through these various stages.

With your first ALERT session, you will probably be at stage zero or one. Gradually, you will relax a little deeper and progress to the next stage. After completing the ALERT program you will have reached stage six.

Using the ALERT is a relaxing and enjoyable experience. Most people forget about the light and sound as they begin to relax deeply. Within seconds, you will probably feel like you've fallen asleep. You will see and hear a rhythm in the form of flashing lights and heartbeat sounds. As you hear and see this rhythm, your brain starts to mirror it. In other words, you become in-synch with the rhythm emitting from the headphone and eye set. With repeated use, your brain learns to practice and master this rhythm.

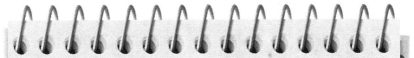

At least six things that happen when you train your brain with the ALERT:

(1) You stimulate and arouse your brain.

(2) You stabilize the tempo of your brainwaves.

(3) You experience a boost of electro-chemical communication in the brain.

(4) You replace your ADHD with the Rhythm of Peak Performance.

(5) You experience an increase in oxygen and blood flow to the brain.

(6) You relax deeply, which lowers stress hormones in the blood (cortisol, adrenaline, and insulin).

If you stick with this program for the next 60 days, then your ADHD symptoms will significantly decrease. Your brain will eventually reorganize itself so that you can concentrate, listen, read, and remember more efficiently.

Bottom line: Just relax and enjoy the process. You can conquer your ADHD while lying flat on your back, with your eyes closed. The only thing you need to do is use your ALERT every day, consistently. Your brain does the rest!

All the best, Nicky

CHAPTER 4

ADHD & The ALERT Brain Training Solution

"Many people feel uncomfortable in the role of the victim of disease. They want a doctor to do something to make them better. The idea of taking a drug to cure a disease seems simpler to accept than the idea of self-healing, And it may be easier for some people. But as researchers recognize the increasingly toxic side effects of many drugs, it is prudent to seek other less intrusive, more natural, often less costly healing techniques." — Barbara Levine (2010), *Your Body Believes Every Word You Say.*

"My daughter uses the ALERT for borderline ADHD. Her teacher uses a checklist to measure ADHD behavior. Before the ALERT, she had a 6 or 7 out of 10 possible check marks for ADHD. After the ALERT, she had a perfect score every day, with no check marks. At home, my husband and I found her to be much more cooperative and less argumentative. Plus, she is doing her homework without bouncing up and down 100 times. For the past two hours, she has been working on her homework without complaining. Unbelievable! One of the biggest changes is her attitude towards us. She realizes right away that she stepped over the line and apologizes almost immediately. Her temper outbursts are almost non-existent." — Karen Rodway, Edmonton. Alberta, Canada.

Suppose you could make a simple shift in your everyday life— which enabled you to read, concentrate, focus, remember and get things done faster than before? Suppose this shift was relatively easy— such as taking a 22 minute nap with headphones and eyeglasses— and that it was safe, deeply relaxing and enjoyable?

The ALERT is a state-of-the-art light and sound machine, with a specific brain training protocol for ADHD. The system has three parts: Eyeglasses, headphones, and a control box with pre-loaded sessions.

The ALERT stands for "Attentive Living through Energizing, Restorative Technology." It is a brain training device that you can use in the comfort of your own home. Actually, you can use the ALERT anywhere. It holds a battery (for portable use) or you can plug it into a wall outlet. It is recommended that you use the ALERT light and sound machine at least once a day, for 60 consecutive days. The device is convenient and easy-to-use and you'll love the way it trains and conditions your brain to get rid of ADHD.

This chapter covers how to use the ALERT, what to expect, and six landmarks to gauge your progress during the 60-day program. In the back of this book, you will also find a handy chart to keep track of your progress.

Development Of The ALERT Light And Sound Machine

The ALERT is the result of 20 years of research, including clinical testing in private schools. The device was developed by school psychologist Michael Joyce and David Siever of Mind Alive Inc.

Joyce & Siever (2001) conducted two clinical studies using light and sound machines to reduce ADHD in elementary school children. The studies showed that specifically-designed light and sound machines reduced ADHD behaviors, such as impulsiveness, inattentiveness, and hyperactivity. Also, the light and sound machines improved the children's reading scores, which reflects an improvement in their ability to concentrate, focus, and retain information.

There is more scientific support for the ALERT technology, but we'll talk about that later. Let's move on to how the device works, so you can get started with your brain training program.

Getting Started With The ALERT

If you've never used a light and sound machine, you're in for a pleasant surprise. It is a soothing, relaxing, and comfortable experience. To prepare, let your friends and family know that you need time alone and shouldn't be disturbed. If possible, mute the ringer on your telephone. You could also put a note on your front door, in case someone drops by unexpectedly. Having a session with the ALERT only takes 22 minutes, so it won't take up too much of your time. After your session, there will be plenty of time to return phone calls and emails, eat dinner, pay your bills, or whatever else you need to do.

How To Use The ALERT

1. **Get comfortable** in a chair or lie down on your bed. You may want to cover yourself up with a blanket.

2. **Put on your ALERT** headphones and eyeglasses.

3. **Power up!** Plug your ALERT into the electrical outlet. (Or use a 9-volt alkaline battery inserted into the back of the device).

4. **Select the setting** that you want on the control box.

5. **Close your eyes**, relax, and enjoy. You will see a pattern of flashing lights, and hear synchronized heartbeat sounds. The rhythm that you're seeing and hearing stimulates and trains your brain to overcome ADHD.

6. **Chill out.** Using the ALERT is so calming and relaxing, that most people enter a state of deep relaxation (which is almost like falling asleep).

7. **You're done!** After 22 minutes, your session is over. You will feel deeply relaxed and energized. Now, you're ready to take charge of your day.

Various Stages Of Deep Relaxation With The ALERT

When you do your first ALERT session, you may wonder what to expect. You may feel tense, frustrated, or restless. You might be telling yourself, "Ok, let's hurry up and get this over with." Or maybe you're anxious about the time, and wondering, "How long is this going to take?" The best thing you can do is go with the flow. Relax and enjoy your ALERT sessions. If this is a new experience for you, it may take a little while to settle down and relax.

You can mentally quiet yourself by focusing on your breathing. Inhale and exhale slowly. Remind yourself, "I'm calm and at ease…. and I just let go." Repeat this phrase silently to yourself: "I just let go… I let go… "

Gentle Awareness

While using the ALERT, it is helpful to have a gentle awareness of your feelings and state of mind. Strive to be calm, peaceful and relaxed. Let things happen in their own time. Be open to the experience. Your thoughts, feelings, and experience may come and go, like leaves floating in a river.

As you use the ALERT, do your best to lie still. Try not to move about. Relax every muscle in your body, from your head to your feet. This will help you to quiet your mind and body.

Biofeedback practitioner Anna Wise (2002) contends that there are six stages (or landmarks) that occur during deep relaxation. When you use the ALERT, you will gradually progress through these various stages. With your first ALERT session, you will probably be at stage zero or one. With each session, you will relax a little deeper and gradually progress to the next stage. After completing the ALERT program you will have reached stage six. Keep in mind that you don't need to experience everything in a particular stage for it to count. You may only experience one or two of the qualities listed. The goal is to reach stage six by the time you complete the ALERT program.

Six Subjective Landmarks For Deep Relaxation

Stage 0:
Mind chatters or inner dialogue (thoughts and cares of the day)
Your thoughts may be rapid and disconnected
A feeling of "Why am I doing this?"
"How much longer is this going to take?"
You may feel restless, frustrated or rushed
Your body is tense

Stage 1:
You're beginning to relax and settle down
Sensation of going under an anesthetic

A feeling of scattered energy
You feel like you're drifting off or being pulled back from the edge of sleep
You may feel dizzy or light headed

Stage 2:
You're starting to feel calm, with flashes of imagery
A feeling of being in between states
You may think back to images from your distant or immediate past
You may have flashbacks from childhood
You may remember traumatic past experiences

Stage 3:
Light, gentle, pleasurable sensations
Mentally stable and calm
More sustained concentration
Very clear mental imagery
Occasional, slight rhythmic movement
May experience the physical sensation of floating, rocking or swaying

Stage 4:
More deeply relaxed than the previous stage
Vivid awareness of breathing, heartbeat or other bodily sensations
Feeling of loss of physical boundaries
Growing very large or very small
Loss of feeling in your hands, feet, legs, or hips
Sensation of being full of air
Sensation of great heaviness or lightness
Alternate between internal and external awareness

Stage 5:
Feeling of being in an altered state peak experience
You have an "aha" experience (light bulb or eureka experience— may only be a brief flash of a split second)
Feeling of deep happiness and satisfaction
Intense alertness, calmness and detachment
Sensation of spacing out or disappearing from the environment or body
Very lucid state of consciousness
May experience extremely vivid imagery

Stage 6:
New way of feeling
Blissful, happy, relaxed, easily letting go, releasing tension and anxiety
Intuitive insight into old problems
Increased awareness about your problems or challenges
Less anxious, angry or frustrated
More relaxed and even-keeled perspective about problems or challenges
A feeling like your old problems are resolved
Whatever you're dealing with, it isn't such a big deal anymore
Perhaps your problem even seems meaningless
It isn't worth getting worked up about it
Sense of understanding of your higher purpose in life

Progressing Through The Stages

As you use the ALERT, you will gradually progress from stages zero to six. There is a big difference between the starting and ending point. You may start out being tense and uptight, but as you continue to use the ALERT, it will become easier and easier to relax.

Stressed Out Versus Relaxed

Consider the difference between being stressed out and relaxed. They are opposite states of mind. Whenever you relax, you release the tension and anxiety. Your body becomes loose, supple, and flexible. This is the opposite of being rigid and uptight. Whenever you "go with the flow," it will be much easier to focus, concentrate and be productive. You also will experience fewer ADHD symptoms.

Less Stress = Less ADHD

You will experience less ADHD symptoms when you're relaxed. At stage six, you will reach a point where you will have an even-keeled perspective about your problems or challenges. You might even realize that whatever you're struggling with is nothing to be worked up about. Perhaps you will let go a little more and resolve to be gentler with yourself, taking things one day at a time.

Another plus of learning to relax is that you'll be able to think sharper, clearer and faster than before. With the ALERT, you'll gradually become a better problem solver. You will explore all your options and implement creative solutions. This is because you tend to think more clearly when you're calm, relaxed and feeling good— versus stressed-out, tense or anxious.

Gauge Your Progress After Your ALERT Session

After your ALERT sessions, refer back to this chapter and ask yourself, "What stage am I at today?" Being aware of your stage (or landmark) will help you to gauge your progress with the ALERT. It gives you a way to describe your experience and recognize what is happening to you. In the back of this book, you will find a bubble chart to record your landmark after each session. Take a few seconds after your ALERT session to reflect upon your experience. Doing this will increase your awareness of the brain training process and help you to recognize the progress that you're making.

How The ALERT Works

The ALERT is a form of audio-visual brain training. Your brain is being stimulated through the ears (auditory cortex) and eyes (visual cortex). Using the ALERT is a relaxing and enjoyable experience. Most people forget about the light and sound as they begin to relax deeply. Within seconds, you will probably feel like you have fallen asleep.

When you use the ALERT, you will see and hear a rhythm in the form of flashing lights and heartbeat sounds. As you hear and see this rhythm, your brain starts to copy and mirror it. In other words, you will become in-synch with the rhythm emitting from the headphone and eye set. With repeated use, your brain learns to practice and master this rhythm.

By training your brain with the ALERT, you will (1) stimulate and arouse the brain, (2) stabilize the tempo of your brainwaves, (3) experience a boost of electro-chemical communication in the brain, (4) replace your ADHD with the Rhythm of Peak Performance, (5) increase oxygen and blood flow to the brain, and (6) relax deeply, which lowers stress hormones in the blood (cortisol, adrenaline, and insulin). We'll be discussing all of these concepts in more detail in the pages to come. The science behind the technology is a little bit complicated, but we will break it down into bite-sized chunks so that it is easier to understand. The ALERT light and sound machine is a home-based brain training program that is safe, reliable, and effective. The technology does all the work for you. It's never been easier to train your brain and transform your life.

The ALERT 60-Day Plan

If you can discipline yourself to use the ALERT at least once a day (for the next 60 days) then you can expect to receive good results.

The ALERT contains 17 pre-programmed sessions. There are 12 protocol sessions, plus an additional 5 sessions (including one for depression).

Five Day Method

You will be doing a total of twelve sessions. It is recommended that you spend five days on each session. Listen to one session for five days and then proceed to the next session. In other words, start with Group A, session A1. Listen to it for five days and then go on to the next session, A2. Listen to it for five days and then go on to the next session, A3. Continue your sessions until you have completed your progress chart. You can also keep track of your sessions in a notebook and journal about your experiences.

When you use the ALERT program, one session a day is the minimum. If you're having a stressful day, you're welcome to do two sessions a day, if you like, but that's optional. The main thing is doing at least one ALERT session every day consistently, for 60 consecutive days.

After you've completed the program, you can use the ALERT occasionally or whenever you feel like it. Many people continue to use their ALERT daily. Of course, the choice is up to you.

It takes only 22 minutes a day to train and condition your mind with the ALERT, and the results are lasting. If you stick with this program for the next 60 days, then your ADHD symptoms will significantly decrease.

Your brain will eventually reorganize itself so that you can concentrate, listen, read, and remember more efficiently.

Here are some aspects of the ALERT program that you'll want to keep in mind:

1. **Practice makes perfect**. When you use the ALERT, you are practicing the Rhythm of Peak Performance. When your brain hears and sees this rhythm, it starts to copy it. This concept is similar to practice, modeling, or training. When you use the ALERT every day, the sights and sounds of the ALERT will create new neural pathways in your brain. You'll notice a gradual improvement in your ability to listen, read, remember, focus, and concentrate.

2. **Expect slow, gradual changes.** You can gauge your progress by noticing your relaxation landmarks, or how you respond to the ALERT sessions. If you feel yourself becoming deeply relaxed while using the ALERT, then you're doing well. Occasionally, there will be days that you may have trouble relaxing, or letting go. Not to worry, you will still benefit from using the ALERT, even if you don't completely relax. Remember that overcoming ADHD is going to take some time. You will experience change in small increments. It takes time to develop the neural circuits in the brain that are necessary for peak performance. Along the way, there will be days where you'll wonder, "Is anything happening at all?" Be patient and keep going with the program. In time, you will see results.

3. **Residual effect.** After using the ALERT, you might feel a buzz. It could be feelings of euphoria, bliss, a burst of energy, or newfound motivation. It is not unusual to experience acute sensory reactions, such as intensified hearing, taste, touch, emotions, or intuition. Some people report that their eyesight sharpens, and things in their room suddenly appear to be more three-dimensional or colorful. This is part of the residual effect. It will stay with you for a while and then usually fades away. It's all part of the training and conditioning process. You may also experience a tingling sensation, in your nose, cheeks, ears, or eyes. It's nothing to worry about, of course. Another usual thing that occasionally happens is a numb feeling in your arms or legs. Again, this is a sign of deep relaxation.

4. **Tension release.** The ALERT will help you to relax so deeply that you may want to sleep for a while. Initially, you will feel sleepy or more tired than usual. If this happens, don't be alarmed. The tension and stress has been stored in your body for a long time, and it's finally being released. When you use the ALERT, you will probably also experience a quick shake of your hand, arm, leg, or foot. It's the same thing that occasionally happens at night, as you drift off to sleep. Again, this is simply the release of tension from the body. It's a normal response and nothing to be concerned about.

5. **Light bulb experiences.** Using the ALERT often results in "Aha!" moments. The deep relaxation provided by the ALERT frees up your creative problem solving side. Sometimes the ALERT removes a mental block—allowing for an instant boost of creativity or flashes of insight. You might come up with new ideas to solve problems that haven't occurred to you before.

6. **Increased awareness.** Many ALERT users report an intense awareness of their body. This is particularly true if you exercise frequently or participate in sports. You may feel your arms, legs or stomach— or experience an intense awareness that is different from the way you usually feel. You may realize that you need to change, or do something differently. Sometimes, we tolerate something for a long time (being overweight, settling for less than we deserve, being in a relationship that isn't working, being messy and disorganized, unfinished projects, etc) and using the ALERT may motivate you to make a change in your life.

How Long Will These Changes Last?

The mental conditioning provided by the ALERT is much like the process of tuning a piano. When the piano is initially tuned, it sounds good for a while, and then it goes back to its old ways. You might wonder, "Why does this piano sound off-key, when it has been professionally tuned?" Of course, the proper tune needs to be conditioned into the piano. The piano needs to be continually readjusted until the proper tone takes root.

It's the same way with the ALERT. You may take two steps forward and then one step back. Be patient with yourself. Each day that you use the ALERT, you are training and conditioning your brain to conquer ADHD.

In time, you will master the new Rhythm of Peak Performance, and this rhythm will eventually replace your old ADHD mindset.

Plateaus. You may hit a plateau with the ALERT program. In other words, you're doing well, but suddenly everything appears to level out. Now it appears that you're staying put rather than progressing to the next level. Plateaus are only temporary. It appears as if no progress is being made, but biological changes are happening internally, in the brain. When you hit a plateau, don't give up. Make some adjustments and keep going until you finish the program.

Unlearning. Using the ALERT will gradually rewire the neural networks in your brain, so that you can focus, concentrate and read better. The rewiring process also includes unlearning the old habits associated with ADHD. Much of this happens on a cellular level. You will slowly gain the capacity to pay attention, focus, and concentrate. It is like getting new shoes— it takes time to get used to the fit, which might be tight at first. Gradually, the contours of your foot will stretch out the shoe and it will seem more natural and comfortable. Take things one day at a time and enjoy the process.

Guardian response. Using the ALERT may bring up old memories, including some painful or embarrassing ones. You may remember something that you haven't thought about in years. The feelings that accompany these memories may be emotionally intense. Don't be afraid or alarmed when these feelings and memories come to the surface. Often, this is part of the healing process. Your reaction may be to guard or protect yourself. However, healing comes when you release and let go with the ALERT sessions.

Consolidation. This is the process where things begin to click and the peak performance mindset becomes refined and automatic. Your brain will have reorganized itself. By the end of 60 days, you will notice a major improvement in your ability to concentrate, focus, get organized, tune out distractions, and get things done. When this happens, your life will be transformed.

Dear Reader,

ADHD experts claim that Ritalin is a magic bullet. They say it's a simple remedy for solving a complex problem. Unfortunately, Ritalin turns out to be a nightmare for most people. It leaves us worse off then before we took the medicine.

When I took Ritalin, I had no idea that it' is an amphetamine (similar to cocaine) and that it could make me crazy, mess up my hormones, stunt my growth, damage my heart, and possibly even kill me. Ritalin's gain isn't worth the pain. It's just not worth it. If you're still not convinced, here are twelve good reasons to avoid Ritalin.

1. Ritalin is a temporary fix, with no long term benefits.

2. If you take Ritalin, you won't experience a long term improvement in your ability to pay attention, concentrate, and focus.

3. Ritalin is a hardcore drug similar to cocaine.

4. Using Ritalin automatically leads to drug addiction.

5. Ritalin causes withdrawal and rebound.

(Continued)

6. Ritalin turns you into a zombie.

7. Ritalin causes Obsessive Compulsive Disorder.

8. Ritalin makes you crazy.

9. Ritalin stunts the growth of children.

10. Ritalin has irreversible side effects, including heart damage.

11. ADHD/Ritalin movement is fueled by the partnership between the APA and drug companies.

12. Ritalin is responsible for deaths and injuries all over the country.

Do these statements seem exaggerated, or couldn't possibly be true? Take a moment to read the next chapter, and consider the facts for yourself.

If you have ADHD, it's only a matter of time before you meet an expert who recommends Ritalin. Perhaps this has already happened to you. Your best defense is to be prepared. You need to know why Ritalin is not the best approach for ADHD. After all, knowledge is power!

All the best,
Nicky

CHAPTER 5

ADHD, Ritalin & "The Emperor's New Clothes"

Do you remember "The Emperor's New Clothes" by Hans Christian Andersen? It's a story about an emperor who is obsessed with his appearance and wardrobe. He hires two experts to make him a new suit. The experts brag that the fabric is invisible to anyone who is stupid or incompetent. The emperor can't see the fabric himself, but pretends that he can, for fear of appearing foolish or unfit for his position. Even the emperor's royal staff agrees that his invisible wardrobe looks stunning. When the emperor parades through town in his invisible clothes, a child cries out, "But, he isn't wearing anything at all!" The emperor cringes, suspecting the assertion is true, but holds his head high. He continues to parade through the streets in his underwear.

It's a clever story, isn't it? On the basis of two experts, the emperor believed that his invisible wardrobe was real. Evidently, the emperor believed the experts on the basis of their authority. Surely, an expert would not lie, deceive, or take advantage. Surely, it would be wise to go along with the experts, rather than look stupid or incompetent. That's why the emperor went against his better judgment. He was afraid of looking stupid, but that's exactly what happened. Wasn't there some pride involved too? The emperor was too proud to admit that he was wrong. He thought it was better to carry on the charade than to admit his mistakes.

What does this story have to do with ADHD? I think the story is a good metaphor for what's happening in the mental health community. The experts who made the invisible coat reminds me of the ADHD/Ritalin advocates. These experts continue to push ADHD drugs on the public, despite overwhelming evidence that Ritalin is dangerous, toxic, and addictive. Unfortunately, the public doesn't have enough information to make an informed decision about Ritalin. Or maybe they have the wrong information.

In his book, *Talking Back To Ritalin*, Dr. Peter Breggin (2001) suggests: "The public has been sold a completely unrealistic picture of Ritalin's value as a treatment. The many professional testimonials about the effectiveness and safety of stimulants are as unreliable as sales pitches for other industrial products that are pushed on consumers" (p. 138).

The ADHD experts praise Ritalin (and other stimulant drugs) as a magic bullet. They say it's a simple remedy for solving a complex problem. The public tends to believe the ADHD/Ritalin advocates, usually on the basis of their authority. Surely, the experts would not lie, deceive, or take advantage. Surely, it would be wise to go along with the experts, because they're acting in our best interest. That's why the public is quick to swallow ADHD pills without doing further research.

Unfortunately, Ritalin turns out to be a nightmare for most people. It leaves us worse off then before we took the medicine. Like an invisible wardrobe, Ritalin turns out to be a fabrication (or deception). The ADHD/Ritalin experts have over-promised and under-delivered. They have betrayed the very people they originally sought to help. Now they must face moral, ethical, legal, and financial consequences.

This is exactly what Psychologist Diane McGuinness maintains in *The Limits Of Biological Treatments For Psychological Distress* (1989):

"The past 25 years has led to a phenomenon almost unique in history. Methodologically rigorous research . . . indicates that ADD and hyperactivity as syndromes simply do not exist. We have invented a disease, given it medical sanction, and now must disown it. The major question is how we go about destroying the monster we have created. It is not easy to do this and still save face" (p. 155).

School Psychologist Michael Valentine declares that Ritalin for ADHD is "one of the biggest frauds ever perpetuated on the educational system, on parents, and on their children. Every medical person involved should be held accountable for it ethically" (Walker, 1998, p. 5).

Neurologist Sidney Walker (1998), in his book *The Hyperactivity Hoax,* contends:

"Doctors who cover up disease symptoms with a feel-good amphetamine drug such as Ritalin are lulling families into believing that their children are being treated when they're merely being pacified by a mind-altering drug, are irresponsible. But an even more irresponsible act being committed by far too many doctors is the drugging of children with no behavior problems at all.

"A few decades ago, boisterous little boys and girls were affectionately called scamps, rascals, and class pests. Now these children are called sick, and doctors are putting them in powerful medications for years or even decades. Doctors are increasingly labeling normal childhood moods and behaviors as hyperactivity and attention disorder and altering these moods and behaviors with potent drugs. In effect, we are coming closer to chemically designing children who will be obedient, docile, and compliant— something that should be abhorrent to moral individuals" (p. 52).

The Ritalin Epidemic: Fueled By Money, Power & Prestige

Unfortunately, most ADHD/Ritalin advocates continue to sing the praises of drugs and DSM-IV, with their heads held high. After all, they have a vested interest in the industry. The ADHD/Ritalin industry is a significant source of income, identity, and authority in the field of pediatrics, family practice, neurology, psychiatry, and pharmacy.

More and more people are being diagnosed with ADHD or ADD, and prescribed drugs. In 2000, it was estimated that five million adults and children were diagnosed with ADHD, and 75-85% of these people were treated with psycho-stimulant medication (CNS Drug Discoveries, 2006).

Obviously, there is a lot of money to be made with ADHD drugs. Global sales of ADHD drugs are forecast to reach $3.3 billion dollars, according to CNS Drug Discoveries. Approximately 97% of these global sales come from the US, with the remainder sold in Europe. The ADHD market is a booming industry, and it's no wonder that ADHD/ Ritalin advocates are stepping up to meet the demand.

Ritalin is widely prescribed, but most doctors are ignorant about how ADHD drugs affect the brain (Breggin, 2002). The average psychiatrist, neurologist, pediatrician and family doctor doesn't know much this either.

Misinformed about Ritalin

There is a tremendous amount of misinformation about ADHD drugs. If you didn't know better, you might think that taking Ritalin is safe and mild, since it is often prescribed to children. Your doctor might tell you that Ritalin washes out of the body in three hours, and has no long term effects. Taking Ritalin is like putting on eyeglasses that sharpen your brain's focus. You might be told that you have a chemical imbalance with ADHD, and Ritalin will fix it. You might be told that you're being irresponsible or negligent if you don't take Ritalin. After all, you've been diagnosed with a psychiatric disorder that requires medical attention.

"Numerous parents have agreed to put their children on Ritalin after doctors hit them with the chronic guilt-provoking line: Depriving your child of Ritalin is like depriving your child of insulin. I've heard this approach so often that I'm starting to wonder if it's being taught in medical school. But I don't care if 100 doctors try this speech on you— Don't fall for it!" (Walker, 1998, p. 55).

"Diabetic children need insulin because their bodies don't produce enough of this necessary hormone. But, as therapist Billy Jay Sahley once said, nobody is suffering from a Ritalin deficiency. Think about it." (Walker, 1998, p. 55).

What's true about Ritalin, and what's not? As always, your best defense is to know the facts. If you have ADHD, it's only a matter of time before you meet an expert who recommends Ritalin. Perhaps this has already happened to you. Your best defense is to be prepared. You need to know exactly why Ritalin is not the best soluton for ADHD. This information will save you time and money. It also protects your well-being.

I'd like you to consider twelve compelling reasons to avoid Ritalin. Equipped with this information, you'll be as wise as the child who cried out, "But, he isn't wearing anything at all!" You'll know better than to waste your time and money on an invisible suit.

Twelve Compelling Reasons To Avoid Ritalin

1. **Ritalin is a temporary fix, with no long term benefits.**
Ritalin works by stimulating and activating the brain. The downside is that it's temporary. It lasts about three to twelve hours, depending on the dose. When the drug wears off, you're right back to where you started. You've put a band-aid on the problem, but the wound is still there. In other words, you are sedated with Ritalin, but not cured. With Ritalin, you merely hide your ADHD symptoms with drugs, and your problems continue.

2. **If you take Ritalin, you won't experience a long term improvement in your ability to pay attention, concentrate and focus.** Neurologist Sidney Walker (1988) contends, "At one time, doctors thought that after a decade or so of Ritalin treatment, behavior-disordered kids would somehow snap out of it and turn into happy, well-adjusted adults. No such luck" (p. 13).

"*Developmental Neurophysiology* notes that clinicians treating large numbers of hyperactive children who were receiving adequate amounts of stimulants and whose medication was well-monitored found that over the years, in spite of medication, many problems continued. By adolescence, these stimulant-treated hyperactive were still failing in school and continued to have behavior problems, many had developed anti-social behaviors, as well as experiencing social ostracism... The children continued to be in various degrees of trouble, and other methods of management as well as (or instead of) stimulants were required" (Walker, 1988, p. 14).

Consider the findings of James Swanson, a widely published psycho-pharmacology researcher and staunch ADHD/Ritalin supporter. Swanson and his team (1993) prepared an Executive Summary for the Department of Education, which contained a comprehensive review of the Ritalin literature based on 300 reviews and 6000 original articles from the last 55 years. Swanson (1993) found:

• Ritalin has no large effects on skills or higher order processes. Teachers and parents should not expect significantly improved reading or athletic skills, positive parenting skills, or learning of new concepts.

• Ritalin has no improvement on long-term adjustment. Teachers and parents should not expect long-term improvement in academic achievement or reduced anti-social behavior.

These dismal findings suggest that Ritalin isn't worth the time, money, or hassle. Ritalin is a temporary fix that only lasts a few hours. It has limited short-term benefit and no long-term value. Any good Ritalin that does immediately disappears once the drug is stopped. Whether you take Ritalin for days, months, or years, your problems will return the day after your last pill is taken (Whalen & Hanker, 1997).

3. **Ritalin is a hardcore drug similar to cocaine.** Ritalin is assumed to be safe and mild because it's often prescribed for children. Some say that Ritalin is a smart drug or cognitive enhancer. In reality, Ritalin (and other ADHD drugs) are pharmacologically similar to cocaine and cause extreme behavioral changes (Rush & Baker, 2001; DEA, 1995).

Almost all ADHD drugs are amphetamines or amphetamine-like stimulants. This includes Ritalin, Daytrana, Equasym and Focalin (methylphenidate), Concerta, Metadate, and Methylin (time-released forms of methylphenidate), Dexedrine and DextroStat (d-amphetamine), Adderall (d-amphetamine and amphetamine mixture), Desoxyn and Gradumet (methamphetamine).

Ritalin is classified with amphetamines in Schedule II by both the Drug Enforcement Agency (DEA) and the International Narcotics Control Board. Evidently, Schedule II indicates the highest possible abuse potential for a prescription drug.

The APA's *Practical Guidelines For The Treatments Of Psychiatric Disorders* (2002) observes that cocaine, amphetamines, and methylphenidate are "neuropharmacologically alike." This textbook points out that abuse patterns are the same for all three drugs. In laboratory tests, people cannot tell the drugs apart in terms of their clinical effects. These drugs can be substituted for each other, and cause similar behavior.

Consider what Dr. Mary Ann Block (2001) says in her book, *No More ADHD*:

"Would you put your children on cocaine to make them sit still, pay attention, and behave? Of course not. But some of you may have done exactly that without even knowing it! The drug in question is Ritalin, which is pharmacologically similar to cocaine. They each go to the same receptor sites in the brain. Ritalin and cocaine are used interchangeably in scientific studies. The DEA has reported this and also states that Ritalin produces cocaine-like effects. The DEA says that taking Ritalin predisposes takers to cocaine's reinforcing effect— a very benign way to say addiction. According to DEA Congressional testimony, neither animals nor humans can tell the difference between cocaine, amphetamines, or methylphenidate (Ritalin) when they are administered the same way in comparable doses. In short, they produce effects that are nearly identical" (Block, 2001).

4. **Using Ritalin automatically leads to drug addiction.** It sets the stage for serious drug abuse. Why? "Because Ritalin isn't curing anything. It isn't even treating anything. Unlike drugs such as insulin or thyroid hormones, Ritalin isn't correcting an identified neurochemical imbalance and thus making the body healthier. It's merely hides the problem for a while, without making the problem go away" (Walker, 1988, p. 35).

"The purpose of Ritalin is to cover up symptoms, much like aspirin masks the pain of a broken leg. When a child stops taking Ritalin, usually in the late teens, the symptoms of the drug has been concealing come back— but the chemical crutch, the daily dose of Ritalin, is gone. It's not surprising that many adolescents seek out a new crutch, any crutch" (Walker, 1988, p. 35).

Ritalin quickly becomes an addiction, an easy way to medicate your symptoms. Self-medicating is a habit that many teens develop when they use Ritalin as children:

"Drugs and alcohol brings them down when they're hyper, calms them when they're anxious, helps them stay alert when they're fatigued, or helps them sleep when they're bothered by insomnia, headaches, dizziness, and other symptoms. It's not a great solution, but it's the only one they've ever known. Ritalin makes kids feel better for a while, But when the kids become teenagers and the prescription for Ritalin stops these individuals turn to other remedies for their pain. The obvious choices: Alcohol and street drugs" (Walker, 1988, p. 40).

What are the warning signs of Ritalin addiction? The major sign is dependency. You're addicted to Ritalin when you cannot function without it, and need it to get through the day. Eventually, a higher dose is needed to get the same effect. "The risk of addiction begins immediately with taking Ritalin as prescribed, and then escalates when and if you develop a tolerance or craving for it" (Breggin, 2001). Even the DEA admits that ADHD drugs can be toxic, and leads to addiction and severe psychological dependence (DEA, 1995).

5. **Ritalin causes withdrawal and rebound.** It's the law of gravity. What goes up must come down. Ritalin makes you high, but you'll come crashing down once the drug wears off. Withdrawal is called "rebound" when you feel worse afterwards than before you took the drug. Breggin (2001) observes:

"Ritalin can cause severe withdrawal symptoms, including crashing with depression, exhaustion, withdrawal, irritability, and suicidal feelings, or excitability, euphoria, and hyperactivity. Psychoses can be precipitated by withdrawal from stimulants. Typically, parents will not recognize a withdrawal reaction when their child gets upset or disturbed after missing even a single dose. They will mistakenly believe their child needs to be put back on the medication or needs more of it" (p. 105).

Yes, Ritalin withdrawal is so powerful that parents think, "Wow, my child must really need this stuff! See how bizarre they behave when the medicine wears off." In reality, your child is angry, crying, depressed, apathetic, or irritable because they're withdrawing (or crashing) as the Ritalin tapers off. With Ritalin, you tend to experience a cycle of energy followed by exhaustion. Rebound is a sign that the body has been harmed and is trying to recuperate (Breggin, 2001).

Rebound symptoms can persist for days after Ritalin has left the body. If you've taken Ritalin for a long time, it may take months for the brain to recover in the absence of the drug (Breggin, 2001).

6. **Ritalin turns you into a zombie.** Remember the zombies from old

black and white movies? With Ritalin, your creativity, spontaneity, and emotional expression fade away. You become glassy-eyed withdrawn, apathetic, isolated, somber, still, and spend time alone. In other words, you've checked out. The lights are on, but nobody's home. It's not a state that you want to be in.

Walker (1988) reported that children respond to Ritalin by becoming "zombie-like, somber, quiet, and still and spend increasing amounts of time alone. If zombification, somberness and social withdrawal are the price a child has to pay for sitting still, that price is too steep" (p. 45).

"While Ritalin makes children sit longer, obey authorities better and complete their homework more easily, it robs children of something more important: Their souls. It makes you feel like you're in an emotional straitjacket. You don't feel like yourself. Your sense of humor is gone" (Walker, 1988, p. 45).

7. **Ritalin causes Obsessive Compulsive Disorder (OCD).**
Ironically, becoming a Ritalin zombie can be mistaken for an improvement. Teachers and parents see it as a good sign when children become more obedient or complaint. They assume subdued behavior equals improved behavior. After all, the child is sitting stoically at their desk, doing their classwork. If the child is at home, they might spend hours and hours drawing, reading, writing, or playing computer games (Breggin, 2001). What parents and teachers may not recognize is that their children have developed OCD symptoms, such as over-erasing, repetitively re-doing, cleaning compulsively (excessive hand washing, showering, or bathing), "checking behaviors" (checking doorknobs, stove, light switches) and lining up their crayons.

While all these symptoms might be interpreted as conscientious, Breggin (2001) insists that drug-induced OCD is a form of severe brain malfunction. He says it isn't a voluntary obsession that a person can stop on their own. OCD enforces social isolation and will not lead to genuine learning. By creating OCD behaviors, Ritalin worsens learning and academic performance, rather than making them better.

Remember how I described my rebound experience in chapter one? My thoughts were stuck in a continuous loop, and I'd check and re-check my schoolwork. I dreamed about doing the same thing over and over. Now, I understand what was happening to me. The pieces finally came together as I was researching and writing this book. These side effects were OCD symptoms!

8. **Ritalin makes you crazy.** If you read the Ritalin warning label, you'll see that "toxic psychosis" is one of the possible adverse effects. This includes hallucinations (seeing things that aren't really there,) recurrent strange ideas, sensations, insecurity or fearfulness, paranoia, and delusions. You can become suspicious, distrustful, imagine things that are unreal, even hallucinate small insects or objects. You can become artificially energized into states of mania, a condition characterized by grandiose plans, bizarre notions of invulnerability, poor judgment, and sometimes paranoia and violence (Breggin, 2001).

For instance, psychiatrist Gerald Young (1981) observed a boy who felt bugs were crawling on him:

"At the time, he complained about mosquitoes, spiders and other bugs, which he thought was getting into his ears, eyes, and nose. He said he could hear the bugs. His methylphenidate (Ritalin) dose during this period ranged from 20 to 30 mg/day. He reported that, "At camp, I saw them—gnats, flies and mosquitoes— they were really true! At the beginning of school, they were really there."

Fortunately, the boy's bug problem stopped when he stopped taking Ritalin. His doctor prescribed Ritalin a second time, but the bug problem immediately returned. The psychiatrist determined the bug problem was an adverse reaction to Ritalin.

9. **Ritalin stunts the growth of children.** Ritalin suppresses appetite and disrupts your growth hormones. The growth suppression involves the entire body and all its organs (Breggin, 2001). For this reason alone, it's a bad idea for children to take ADHD drugs.

10. **Ritalin has irreversible side effects, including heart damage.** ADHD drugs cause your veins and arteries to squeeze together (or contract) so that your heart works overtime. This adverse reaction is listed in the *Physician's Desk Reference* (2010). The side effects inevitably

leads to heart damage. Even if you don't have preexisting heart problems, medical researchers suggest that Ritalin may cause sudden death (Kuehn, 2009; Gould & Walsh, 2009).

11. **ADHD/Ritalin movement is fueled by the partnership between the APA and drug companies.** The push towards Ritalin (and other ADHD drugs) is driven by money. It's a lucrative drug with a high profit potential. Money is the bottom line. That's why drugs are touted as the best treatment for ADHD, despite evidence to the contrary.

I highly recommend that you read Psychiatrist Peter Breggin's book *Talking Back To Ritalin: What Doctors Aren't Telling You About Stimulants And ADHD*. Most of this chapter is based on Breggin's book. He is known as the "Ralph Nader of psychiatry," and has written several books on the use and misuse of psychoactive medications. He has also served as a medical expert in multiple court cases on this subject.

Breggin (2001) claims that the ADHD/Ritalin movement is fueled by a partnership between the APA and the pharmaceutical industry. Here is the amazing story of how this happened, which I've paraphrased from Breggin's book.

In the 1970s, the DSM was revised, so that psychological diagnoses would sound more medical. ADHD was established to be an official mental disorder that was best treated with drugs. At the same time, the APA was barely making ends meet. Psychiatrists were at the bottom of the medical income scale. They also faced stiff competition from other mental health professionals such as psychologists, social workers, counselors. and therapists. To promote psychiatry, they used the DSM to convince the public that psychological problems are rooted in genetics and biology, and required drug treatment.

At the time, the APA did not have the financial resources to rewrite and publicize the Diagnostic Manual. In order to raise capital, the APA created a partnership with drug companies. The partnership would enable psychiatry to use drug company funds to promote the medical model, psychopharmacology. The partnership also established psychiatry as an expert authority, with a powerful influence on mental health and medicine. Backed by the multi-billion dollar drug industry, psychiatry sought to be more powerful than non-medical professionals, such as psychologists and social workers. Within a few years, the APA transformed itself from a failing institution into one of the most powerful political forces in the nation. The APA also developed lobby groups in state capitals and Washington, DC to gain a stronger influence in the media and the courts, and to distribute drugs to greater numbers of people. Even CHADD (Children and Adults with Attention Deficit Disorder,) a support group formed in 1987, received substantial financial support from Ciba Geneva Pharmaceuticals, the manufacturer of Ritalin (Breggin, 2001).

Evidently, the medical credo of, "First, do no harm," has been replaced with the marketing credo of "sell, sell, sell!" (Adams, 2008).

12. **Ritalin is a prescription for countless tragedies.** ADHD drugs are responsible for an endless stream of deaths and injuries all over the country. Consider the following case studies:

May, 2009. John was wrongly prescribed Risperdal, an anti-psychotic medication, for ADHD at age 7. The drug made him aggressive, sleepy, and constipated. As a result of taking Risperdal, John also grew breasts (which made him look like a girl). His parents launched a class action lawsuit against the drug manufacturer for fraud. John stopped taking the drugs, but his chest did not return to normal. At age 19, he needed plastic surgery to restore his chest to its normal size. In fact, John needed a double mastectomy, and he continues to have health problems (CBS News, 2009).

February, 2007. FDA requested that ADHD drug companies develop "Patient Medication Guides" to warn users about cardiovascular risks and adverse psychiatric symptoms associated with their medicines (FDA News Release, 2007).

February, 2005. In Canada, 14 children and six adults died after taking the recommended dose of Adderall. The drug was taken off the market, but reintroduced six months later (FDA 2005 & DeNoon 2005).

June, 2005. FDA reported that Concerta (and other methylphenidate drugs) caused psychotic behavior, hallucinations, suicidal tendencies, aggression, and violent behavior. The FDA promised to make safety warnings labels, as required by the Best Pharmaceutical for Children Act (FDA Advisory Committee, 2005).

September, 2005. The FDA issued a Public Health Advisory warning that children and adolescents being treated with the ADHD drug Strattera should be closely monitored for suicidal thinking or behaviors (FDA Public Health Advisory, 2005).

October, 2005. The FDA withdrew the ADHD drug Cylert because it causes liver problems, including death. The FDA concluded that the overall risk of liver toxicity from these ADHD drugs outweigh the benefits (FDA Public Health Advisory, 2005).

December, 2004. The FDA requires Strattera to post a warning label that it may cause severe liver damage, progressing to liver failure, and resulting in death. The labeling came after two reports that a teenager and adult suffered liver damage while using Strattera (FDA Talk Paper T04-60, 2004).

February, 2001. Shaina Dunkle, age 10, died after taking Ritalin for two years in McKean County, Pennsylvania. The medical examiners concluded that the main cause of death was toxicity. Her body was not excreting the drug properly and was building up a toxic amount until she went into cardiac arrest (Dunkle, 2010).

April, 2000. Matthew Smith, age 14, collapsed at his home while playing with a skateboard and was later pronounced dead at a hospital. The medical examiner in Pontiac, Michigan concluded that the boy died of a heart attack, most likely caused by ten years of taking Ritalin for ADHD. At autopsy, Matthew's heart showed clear signs of small vessel damage. His death certificate reads, "Death caused from long term use of Methylphenidate, Ritalin." Matthew's parents said they were pressured to put their child on Ritalin because the school threatened to report them to Child Protective Services for medical negligence if they did not do so. The parents reluctantly put their child on the drug which the medical examiner says ultimately killed him (Sightings, 2000; Block 2001).

January, 1999. Ryan Ehlis, a college student in Bismarck, North Dakota, took Adderall to control his ADHD. Ten days later, he slipped into a psychotic fog and killed his infant twin daughters. He said that God told him to do it. The courts found him innocent after testimony by a psychiatrist and the drug manufacturer said his psychotic state was a very rare side effect of Adderall (Musca, 2009; Jones 2008).

April, 1999. Shawn Cooper, a 15-year-old-sophomore at Notus Junior-Senior High School in Notus, Idaho, was taking Ritalin when he fired two shotgun rounds, narrowly missing students and school staff. He shot and injured one student and held the school hostage for 20 minutes. Terrified students ran for their lives, and barricaded themselves in classrooms (Pringle, 2006).

May, 1999. T. J. Solomon, a 15-year-old at Heritage High School in Conyers, Georgia, was being treated with Ritalin when he opened fire on and wounded six classmates (CNN News, 1999).

March, 1998. Andrew Golden, age 11, and Mitchell Johnson, age 14, opened fire in a high school in Jonesboro, Arkansas. They shot 15 people, killing four students, one teacher, and wounding 10 others. Both boys had been diagnosed with ADD and prescribed Ritalin prior to the shooting (Indystar, 2006; Clifton, 1998).

May, 1998. Kip Kinkel, 15-year-old sophomore at Thurston High School in Springfield, Oregon, murdered his parents. After the murder, he went to school and opened fire on students in the cafeteria, killing two and wounding 22 teenagers. Kip was taking both Ritalin and Prozac (Verhovek, 1999; Skrzypek, 2010).

May, 1997. Jeremy Strohmeyer, age 18, sexually-assaulted and murdered a 7-year-old girl in Las Vegas, Nevada. He had been diagnosed with ADD and prescribed Dexedrine prior to the killing (New York Times, 1988).

December, 1997. Michael Carneal, age 14, opened fire on students at a high school prayer meeting in West Paducah, Kentucky. At the time, he had been diagnosed with ADD and was taking Ritalin. Three teenagers were killed, four others were wounded, and one student was paralyzed (Newman, 2007).

January, 1996. Stephanie Hall, age 12, died in her sleep from cardiac arrhythmia. She had been taking Ritalin for five years, and often complained about stomachaches and nausea. She also displayed mood swings and bizarre behavior (Baughman, 1998).

ADHD Drugs Responsible For Countless Deaths & Injuries

The internet, newspapers and TV are flooded with horror stories about the aftermath of ADHD drugs. Even government agencies (such as the DEA and FDA) list hundreds of ADHD-related deaths and injuries. Sadly, this represents a gross understatement of statistics. The truth is that the ADHD drugs are responsible for an endless stream of deaths and injuries all over the country.

How tragic that ADHD drugs have claimed so many victims. These people did not deserve the fate they received. If only they could go back in time, and try brain training instead of Ritalin. My friend, it's too late for these victims, but it's not too late for you. There has never been a better time to train your brain and transform your life.

I'd like to end this chapter with an excerpt from *The Harm Reduction Guide To Coming Off Psychiatric Drugs* (2007). Author Will Hall, Founder of the Massachusetts-based Freedom Center, shares from his own experience:

"I used many different psychiatric drugs over several years, but the medical professionals who prescribed them never made me feel empowered or informed. They didn't explain how the drugs work, honestly discuss the risks involved, offer alternatives, or help me withdraw when I wanted to stop taking them. Information I needed was missing, incomplete, or inaccurate. When I finally began to learn ways to get better without medication, it wasn't because of the mental heath system, it was in spite of it.

"Part of me didn't really want to be on psychiatric drugs, but another part of me desperately needed help. My suffering was very serious: Multiple suicide attempts, hearing persecutory voices, extreme mistrust, bizarre experiences, hiding alone in my apartment, unable to take care of myself. Therapy hadn't worked, and no one offered me other options. I was under pressure to see my problems as biologically-based and needing medication, instead of looking at medication as one option among many. For a time, medication seemed like my only way out. It took years to learn that the answers, and my hope for getting better, were really within myself.

"When I finally left the hospitals, residential facilities, and homeless shelters that I lived in for nearly a year, I began to do my own investigating. I started judging my options more carefully, not based on misinformed authorities telling me what to do, but on my own research and learning. That process led me to co-found Freedom Center, a support community in Western Massachusetts that brings together people asking similar questions.

"Through the Freedom Center, I discovered that I was denied a basic medical right: Informed consent, having accurate information about my diagnosis and medication. I learned that mistreatment like I went through is business as usual in the mental health profession. I came across research ignored by the mainstream media, including studies by the UK charity MIND and the British Psychological Society, which confirmed my experience. Most professionals are not only ignorant about coming off drugs, but frequently stand in patients' way, sometimes ending up harming them.

"Many of us are living without psychiatric drugs that the doctors told us we would need our whole lives, and despite (my) diagnosis… I have been medication-free for more than 13 years."

No "Magic Bullet" For ADHD

What a powerful testimony of recovering from psychoactive medication. There is a popular slogan which suggests, "Just say no to drugs." That's good advice. Remember the story of the "Emperor's New Clothes." The experts claim that Ritalin is a magic bullet, but it's really nothing more than an invisible suit. Personally, I fell into this trap when I took Ritalin. I was like that foolish emperor who accepted the advice of experts, and put on an invisible suit. I had no idea that Ritalin was an amphetamine (similar to cocaine) and that it could make me crazy, mess up my hormones, stunt my growth, damage my heart, and possibly even kill me. Ritalin's gain isn't worth the pain. It's just not worth it.

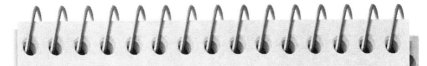

Dear Reader,

Ritalin's gain isn't worth the pain, but I always wondered why the drug works. How does Ritalin eliminate the symptoms of ADHD, if only temporarily? Also, is there a natural remedy that works like Ritalin, without the awful side effects?

I read everything that I could find about Ritalin, and talked to local pharmacists. I discovered that Ritalin is a powerful stimulant. It wakes up, stimulates and arouses the brain. Ritalin also boosts neurotransmitters (dopamine) in the brain, and speeds up slow brainwaves.

There are at least three causes for ADHD:

(1) Neurotransmitter deficiency (or disruption)
(2) Slow brainwaves
(3) Low arousal

The good news is that Ritalin addresses all three things. The bad news is that Ritalin also negates the benefits and makes the problem worse.

Ritalin wreaks havoc with brain chemistry and structure, which can clearly be seen on brain scans.

(Continued)

Ritalin floods the brain with dopamine, which results in the depletion and deregulation of dopamine as well as other neurotransmitters involved in stress and reward.

Ultimately, Ritalin covers up the symptoms of ADHD, much like aspirin masks the pain of a broken leg. If you have a broken leg, you can take aspirin to numb the pain, but it isn't doing anything to heal your leg. It's the same thing with Ritalin.

Having ADHD is like sitting on a tack. You could take medicine for relief, but the best treatment is removing the tack. If you want to get to the root of the problem, once and for all, grab that tack and pull it out. Whew, doesn't that feel better now?

With brain training, you can pull the tack out. You can stimulate and activate your brain, and get the positive results of Ritalin, without swallowing pills. Isn't that good news? If you'd like to know more, be sure to read the next chapter.

All the best,
Nicky

CHAPTER 6

Three Ways That Ritalin
Stimulates And Arouses The Brain

My personal experience with Ritalin is something that I wouldn't wish on my worse enemy. The medicine works wonders, but it's a nightmare once it wears off. Coming down from Ritalin is like taking a sharp drop on a roller coaster ride. It reminds me of a ride that loops upside down and goes backwards in the dark. After a while, it isn't fun anymore. Taking Ritalin can be a scary experience. When I stopped taking Ritalin, I read everything that I could find about ADHD, neuroscience and brain power. I always wondered why Ritalin works. How does Ritalin eliminate the symptoms of ADHD, if only temporarily? Also, is there a natural remedy that works like Ritalin, without the awful side effects?

In the midst of my research, I stumbled upon the scientific premise behind Ritalin. Once I understood how and why Ritalin worked, I realized that the same thing could be accomplished with brain training.

To my surprise, there are many books and journal articles that advocate brain training instead of drugs, and they're written by medical doctors, neuroscientists, psychologists and psychiatrists (Bragin, 2007; Doidge, 2007; Fernandez & Goldberg, 2009; Gimpel, 2007; Kawashima, 2004, 2008; Steinberg & Othmer, 2004; Swingle, 2008; Hill & Castro, 2002, 2009).

There is a small scientific community who recommends brain training instead of Ritalin. Even the *Scientific American* suggests that brain training for ADHD may be just as effective as stimulant medication, but that this approach requires more patience and effort (Sinha, 2005).

Consider what psychiatrist and neurologist Ammon Gimpel (2007) says in his book, *Brain Exercises To Cure ADHD*:

"The difficulty with ADHD is that, despite being recognized more easily by professionals in recent years, most physicians and therapists do not have a long-term solution. Medication, such as Ritalin, cannot solve the problems associated with ADHD alone, nor does it result in any permanent changes in the brain. As soon as the Ritalin is stopped, the symptoms of ADHD return. Now, however, new techniques and strategies, targeted mental and physical exercises have proven to reduce and permanently eliminate the symptoms of ADHD in children, teenagers and adults.... The research that has been done in the last few years will have a profound effect on how we treat memory loss, learning disabilities, psychological difficulties, ADHD, brain injury and a host of other disabilities. If the Nobel Prize is based on the number of people whose quality of life will be greatly improved, then this revolutionary breakthrough in brain physiology will be worthy of one" (p. 3 - 4).

Three Ways That Ritalin Stimulates The Brain

How can you train your brain, and get the positive results of Ritalin, without swallowing pills? To answer this question, let's look at three ways that Ritalin stimulates and activates the brain.

1. **Ritalin boosts neurotransmitters in the brain.** It's commonly believed that ADHD is the result of a chemical imbalance in the brain (Monastra, 2005). Whenever experts talk about a chemical imbalance, they're always referring to neurotransmitters. It's explained in more detail in the next chapter, but neurotransmitters refer to brain chemicals such as dopamine, serotonin, norepinephrine, and endorphins. Neuro-transmitters are chemical messengers that enable your brain cells (or neurons) to talk to each other. Neurotransmitters determine your moods, memory and behavior.

Researchers have found that ADHD is caused by a disruption or deficiency of neurotransmitters in the brain (Volvow, Wang, & Kollins, 2009). Ritalin works by boosting neurotransmitters in the brain, so that you can pay attention, concentrate, focus, and tune out distractions (Gottlieb, 2001, Volkow 2001).

2. **Ritalin speeds up slow brainwaves.** Researchers have found that folks with ADHD have slower brainwaves than normal people (Lubar,

Swartwood, Swartwood & O'Donnell, 1995; Lubar 1984, 1991). ADHD brainwaves tend to be slow and sluggish, which causes you to become easily distracted. This is why your brain turns off when things are boring, uninteresting, overly complicated, or hard to understand. When something doesn't arouse your attention, you mentally shut down and tune out. Ritalin works by speeding up slow brainwaves, which makes it easier for you to read, write, remember, and get your work done.

3. **Ritalin boosts arousal in the brain.** Researchers say that ADHD is caused by low arousal (Satterfield & Dawson, 1971; Satterfield & Lasser, 1973; Gray & Amen 2003, Monastra, 2005) or the brain not getting enough stimulation. In other words, your brain craves some extra stimulation, so that you can get into gear. That's why you're often bored, and tend to procrastinate. With ADHD, you have a sleepy brain. Ritalin works by increasing the brain's physiological arousal so that you can pay attention, focus, and concentrate.

Suppose you're tapping your feet, doodling on paper, feeling anxious or frustrated about something, or struggling with restless energy. Do you really need more stimulation? Yes, stimulation is exactly what you're craving. It seems ironic, but you're restless because you're not getting enough stimulation. This is exactly what happens when you're bored. You aren't experiencing enough arousal or stimulation to pique your interest. That's why you try to get yourself up (or aroused) by drinking coffee, energy drinks, or taking drugs. You might even try thrill-seeking activities, picking a fight, or causing some commotion. You're attempting to get yourself up or aroused. Low arousal refers to how sleepy or awake the brain is. People with ADHD tend to have low states of arousal, and seek new stimulation to get themselves up.

In the late 70s and early 80s, psychologists called this the Low Arousal Theory—and it was generally accepted in the medical community as a driving force behind ADHD, as it remains today (Hill & Castro, 2002). This is why Ritalin has a profound effect on ADHD. It boosts low levels of arousal and wakes up the brain so you can focus, pay attention, and get things done.

Interestingly, your brain can be over-aroused or under-aroused. Either way, your brain isn't functioning optimally. If your brain is over-aroused, you might be wired, jumpy, hyperactive, or anxious. You might be trying to do too much, or feel overwhelmed. If your brain is under-aroused, then you will probably feel sleepy, lethargic, bored, or apathetic. You may not care or be aware of what is happening around you. Your restlessness can be an unconscious, automatic behavior trying to wake up your brain (Hill & Castro, 2002).

To recap, there are at least three causes for ADHD: Neurotransmitter deficiency or disruption, slow brainwaves, and low arousal. The good news is that Ritalin addresses all three things. The bad news is that Ritalin also negates these benefits and makes the problem worse.

Neurotransmitter Deficiency Worsens With Ritalin

"ADHD/Ritalin advocates frequently claim that Ritalin enhances or improves nerve transmission in the brain by correcting biochemical imbalances. These are unfounded speculations aimed at justifying the use of medication. *Instead of improving brain function, Ritalin and other stimulants create severe biochemical imbalances.* They do not normalize the brain. They render it abnormal. This cannot be overemphasized. Stimulants produce pathological malfunctions in the child's brain. Whenever the drugs have any direct effect on the child's mind or behavior, they do so by disrupting brain function. The effective doses of Ritalin, Adderall, and similar drugs always cause malfunctions in the brain" (Breggin, 2001, p. 81).

Ironically, Ritalin worsens the very problem that it attempts to correct: Neurotransmitter deficiency. With Ritalin, your brain assumes it has an abundance of neurotransmitter chemicals, such as serotonin and dopamine. In reality, Ritalin artificially boosts the brain's level of serotonin and dopamine, and your brain assumes everything is fine—so that it doesn't need to produce any more neurotransmitters. As a result, your brain gets lazy. Your brain assumes that it can sit back and take it easy. After all, there are more than enough neurotransmitters to go around. Eventually, your brain's natural supply of neurotransmitters is depleted or used up. When this happens, you may experience serious psychiatric symptoms, such as depression and anxiety (Hinz, 2010a). What has happened is that the brain's regulatory mechanisms have been altered. The brain is no longer manufacturing neurotransmitters on its own. Now, you will need to take more Ritalin in order to return to normal chemical levels in the brain. In other words, you're dependent upon Ritalin to function. You can't go without it anymore. You crave Ritalin, and it's intensified by your dependency and addiction to the drug. Ironically, Ritalin worsens the very problem that it seeks to correct. In the long run, Ritalin perpetuates neurotransmitter deficiency, rather than correcting it (Hinz, 2010b).

Slow Brainwaves Worsen With Ritalin

With Ritalin, your brainwaves are subjected to an up-and-down roller coaster ride. Ritalin artificially speeds up your brainwaves, but later you'll come crashing down when the medicine wears off. It's the rebound effect and it includes depression, loss of energy, feelings of overwhelm, and anxiety. You might be tempted to take more Ritalin to cope with these feelings, but then you're too wired to settle down and sleep. Your brainwaves quickly become dependent on Ritalin to speed up. Your brainwaves rely on Ritalin for an instant artificial boost. Over time, your brainwaves become more and more sluggish. In fact, your brain gets to the point that it can't function without Ritalin. That's when tolerance kicks in and a stronger dose is needed to get the same effect. Once again, Ritalin worsens the problem (slow brainwaves) rather than making it better.

Low Arousal Worsens With Ritalin

With ADHD, you tend to be restless and easily bored. Don't you hate that feeling? You're struggling with low energy, and can't seem to get into gear, when you have so many things to do. Well, feeling sluggish is bad, but being wired is worse. Your brain is running on speed with Ritalin. Over time, Ritalin makes you toxic. Your veins and arteries squeeze together so that your heart works overtime. This inevitably leads to heart damage and toxicity. Over time, it becomes more and more difficult to raise your energy level. Your brain gets lazy, because it is dependent upon an artificial stimulant to get you energized. Typically, when Ritalin stops working, doctors do one of the following: (1) increase the dose of the drug, (2) switch to another drug, or (3) add a second drug. All three of these things do nothing to address the problem that caused the drug to stop working and simply sets up conditions that cause more problems (Hinz, 2010b).

Having ADHD Is Like Sitting On A Tack

Ritalin covers up the symptoms of ADHD, much like aspirin masks the pain of a broken leg. If you have a broken leg, you can take aspirin to numb the pain, but it isn't doing anything to heal your leg. It's the same thing with Ritalin. It's like sitting on a tack. You could take medicine for relief, but the best treatment is removing the tack. If you want to get to the root of the problem, once and for all, grab that tack and pull it out. Whew, doesn't that feel better now?

With brain training, you can pull the tack out. You can stimulate and activate your brain, and get the positive results of Ritalin, without swallowing pills. Isn't that good news? Let's take a look at how this works.

Neurotransmitter Deficiency

The ALERT uses the Sensory Motor Rhythm to stimulate and arouse your brain. The gentle rhythmic stimulation provokes your brain cells to wire and fire correctly, produce a stable supply of neurotransmitters, and successfully connect to neighboring neurons at the synapse. The ALERT also increases oxygen and blood flow to the brain. The ALERT does this with gentle light and sound stimulation to the visual cortex and auditory cortex. As a result, your brain naturally compensates for any neurotransmitter deficiency or disruption that it may be experiencing.

Slow Brainwaves

With ADHD, your brainwaves tend to be slow or sluggish. You're like a person who is flabby, weak, and out-of-shape. The solution is not drugs, but rather training your brain.

Using the ALERT stimulates, conditions, and exercises your brainwaves. With repeated practice, your brainwaves become steady, even-keeled and balanced. By using the ALERT, you speed up the slow brainwaves of ADHD with the Rhythm of Peak Performance, or Sensory Motor Rhythm. It is a rhythm that is scientifically proven to help you conquer ADHD, so that you can concentrate, focus, and remember.

Low Arousal In The Brain

The ALERT's Sensory Motor Rhythm also boosts your arousal level. The audio-visual stimulation naturally turns on your brainpower, and flips the switch on your brain's arousal. You'll receive just the right amount of stimulation—not too much that you'll feel wired, jumpy, or anxious—and not too little that you feel lethargic, bored or apathetic. The ALERT gently boosts your arousal levels, so that your brain functions optimally.

As mentioned previously, the ALERT also increases oxygen and blood flow to the brain, which enables you to think faster on your feet. You'll also have a higher threshold for stress, so that you're more flexible (rather than rigid,) easy going and calm (rather than tense and uptight,) plus you're focused and organized (rather than distracted and scattered). With the ALERT brain training program, you'll experience a burst of energy that enables you to face any challenges that come your way.

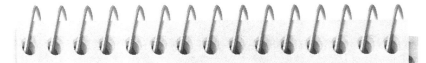

Dear Reader,

It's a controversial subject, but sometimes ADHD is described as a chemical imbalance. What does that mean? Evidently, certain chemicals are deficient or lacking in the brain. How do you test a person for chemical imbalances? If you look in the DSM-IV, it says nothing about chemical imbalances.

While researching this book, I finally found some answers. A chemical imbalance refers to a deficiency or disruption of neurotransmitters in the brain. Researchers have found that ADHD sufferers have a deficiency of the neurotransmitter dopamine.

Did you know that independent laboratories can test your neurotransmitter levels, based on a urine sample? Evidently, neurotransmitters are present in many body fluids, including saliva, urine, cerebral spinal fluid, and serum (Ailtis & Ailtis, 2007). Scientists have established a normal (or healthy) range for various neurotransmitters. Anything out-of-range (above or below the standard range) is considered to be abnormal levels of neurotransmitters.

Evidently, neurotransmitter testing falls under the umbrella of forensic pathology.

(Continued)

Testing for neurotransmitters is a specialized test, and you must request it from an outside lab. Unfortunately, doctors rarely (if ever) test a person's neurotransmitter levels before making a diagnosis of ADHD or ADD. It's just not a common practice.

Plus, it's not an official ADHD test. The link between dopamine deficiency and ADHD has been reported in scientific journals, but the DSM-IV says absolutely nothing about chemical imbalances or neurotransmitter levels.

The next chapter reveals how the so-called chemical imbalance of ADHD can be corrected by eating dopamine-rich foods for optimum brain health.

"Until recently, the idea that food might profoundly and rapidly influence brain chemistry was considered scientifically ludicrous...(but) it turns out that the brain is uniquely responsive to food chemicals," writes Jean Carper (2000), in her book Your Miracle Brain (p. 9).

Want to know more? Be sure to read the next chapter.

All the best,
Nicky

CHAPTER 7

Demystifying The Chemical Imbalance Of ADHD

"ADHD is caused by the abnormal functioning of neurotransmitters, the chemical messengers of the brain. It looks very much like a willpower problem, but it isn't. It's essentially a chemical problem in the management systems of the brain. Serotonin and dopamine are examples of neurotransmitters. When neurotransmitters become balanced, the negative symptoms diminish. Neurotransmitter therapy is a natural ADHD treatment. ADD and ADHD are conditions that can be easily corrected without drugs, enabling you to live a fulfilled and successful life." —Dr. Ross Stewart (2011), founder of NeuroWellness.

The concept of ADHD being a chemical imbalance is somewhat overwhelming and scary, isn't it? It doesn't have to be like that. A chemical imbalance is just a fancy label for the deficiency or disruption of certain brain chemicals. This chapter attempts to explain and demystify the ADHD chemical imbalance concept, and offer some nutritional tips for bringing the mind and body into equilibrium.

Researchers claim that ADHD is caused by a deficiency of dopamine, a brain chemical (or neurotransmitter) that helps us to focus and concentrate (Gottlieb, 2001; Volkow, Wang & Fowler, 2001; Volkow, Wang & Kollins, 2009).

What Reduces Our Natural Supply Of Neurotransmitters?

The brain produces neurotransmitters that are critical to every thought and feeling that we experience. We typically have sufficient levels of neurotransmitters until we experience a crisis, trauma, or stressful disruption. That's when we experience a deficiency or disruption of neurotransmitters, which leads to problems with distraction— which is typical of ADHD. A crisis reduces our brain's reserves of neurotransmitters, such as serotonin, dopamine or norepinephrine.

Interestingly, neurotransmitter deficiency (or disruption) has been linked to depression, schizophrenia, Alzheimer's Disease, anxiety disorders, Obsessive Compulsive Disorder, and social phobias. It all starts with neurotransmitter problems in the brain.

How My Psychology Professor Explained Chemical Imbalances

When I attended university, I took an "Abnormal Psychology" class. My professor worked in a mental institution, and often talked about chemical imbalances in the brain. He said that all psychiatric illness results from chemical imbalances in the brain. My professor suggested that some people are born with a chemical imbalance; other times it happens as a result of a crisis.

Evidently, a person's response to a crisis makes all the difference. My professor explained that a crisis brings out strong emotions, such as self-pity, panic, anguish, anger, or fear. If these emotions spiral out of control, it may be difficult to bounce back, and return to the way things were before. It may be a struggle to go back to work or school, or even take care of yourself.

Consider a healthy man who becomes depressed when his wife dies. He is so upset that he can't sleep or eat. He doesn't feel like doing anything. He lies in bed all day and watches TV. He feels lonely, and his internal dialogue becomes negative and self-defeating. The man loses interest in grooming, bathing, cooking, cleaning, and working. He stops taking care of himself, and his life falls apart. His emotions spiral out of control, and his internal chemistry becomes unbalanced. As a result, the man develops severe depression.

My professor explained that chemical imbalances are commonly blamed for ADHD and ADD. Sometimes, a crisis (such as a divorce or death of a family member) can trigger symptoms of ADHD. This crisis would make things difficult for a child to concentrate and focus in school. A crisis is also stressful for adults, and may affect work performance, relationships, and outlook on life.

Testing Neurotransmitter Levels

Did you know that independent laboratories can test your neurotransmitter levels, based on a urine sample? Evidently, neurotransmitters are present in many body fluids, including saliva, urine, cerebral spinal fluid, and serum (Ailtis & Ailtis, 2007).

Scientists have established a normal (or healthy) range for various neurotransmitters. Anything out-of-range (above or below the standard range) is considered to be abnormal levels of neurotransmitters. Low levels of neurotransmitters are commonly considered to be a chemical imbalance.

Although neurotransmitter testing is fairly straight-forward, there are at least four pitfalls when it comes to chemical imbalances.

Four Pitfalls About Testing For Chemical Imbalances:

(1) **Willy-nilly labeling.** Often, the assessment of a chemical imbalance is made intuitively, which raises red flags. It isn't fair (or accurate) to label someone with a chemical imbalance when they haven't been tested. As previously mentioned, the validity of the DSM-IV check list for ADHD, various ADHD questionnaires, and computer-based testing for ADHD has also been questioned, because it is so subjective. The use of a neurotransmitter test to measure dopamine levels for ADHD seems to be a step in the right direction, when it comes to making an objective assessment. This way, a person can know exactly which brain chemicals are low or deficient, and take the proper steps to correct the problem.

(2) **Neurotransmitter testing is rarely (if ever) offered.** Neurotransmitter testing falls under the umbrella of forensic pathology. It's a specialized test, and you'd have to request it from an outside lab. Unfortunately, doctors rarely (if ever) test a person's neurotransmitter levels before making a diagnosis of ADHD or ADD. It's not a common practice.

(3) **It's not an official ADHD test.** The link between dopamine deficiency and ADHD has been reported in scientific journals (Gottlieb, 2001; Volkow, Wang & Fowler, 2001; Volkow, Wang & Kollins, 2009).

However, the DSM-IV says absolutely nothing about chemical imbalances or neurotransmitter levels.

(4) **Pills are wrongly considered to be chemical balancers.**

Ritalin and other ADHD drugs numb and cover up the pain, but do not make any lasting, healthy changes in the brain. It's better to explore natural ways to bring the brain into balance, such as brain training, eating nutritious food, and exercising.

Psychiatrist Daniel Amen (2002) contends that ADHD is caused by neurotransmitter deficiencies as well as specific parts of the brain being overactive or underactive. He makes assessments using SPECT brain scans, brain imaging, and genetic research. Dr. Amen uses these measures to diagnose and verify ADHD. In his various books, such as *Healing ADD* (1999) and *The Mars And Venus Diet And Exercise Solution* (2003, co-authored with John Gray), Dr. Amen recommends eating "brain healthy foods" and other natural ways to overcome neurotransmitter deficiencies or chemical imbalances.

ADHD & Neurotransmitter Deficiency

The main neurotransmitter blamed for ADHD is dopamine. This "feel good" neurotransmitter is part of the reward system in the brain. Dopamine regulates movement, thought, and behavior (Volkow, Wang & Kollins, 2009). Your brain releases dopamine whenever you're rewarded, even if it's simply with a nod, handshake, pat on the back, or someone says, "Good job!" Your brain releases dopamine whenever you receive positive feedback. Dopamine makes you feel happy and euphoric.

At least three neurotransmitters influence your ability to learn: Dopamine, acetylcholine, and norepinephrine. Dopamine plays a big role in what you're able to remember. Dopamine takes images and concepts that are temporarily stored in your short-term memory, and moves them into your long-term memory. Dopamine converts new knowledge into long-term or permanent knowledge (Johnson & Trivitayakhun, 2010).

Low dopamine levels can cause depression, dissatisfaction, addictions, cravings, compulsions, low sex drive, as well as an inability to focus (Turcotte, 2010).

A study conducted by the U.S. Department of Energy's Brookhaven National Laboratory in New York State found that ADHD sufferers have deficiencies in the way the brain deals with dopamine, the neurotransmitter which elicits feelings of pleasure and is naturally released in rewarding experiences (Volkow, Wang & Kollins, 2009).

Researchers also claim that low dopamine is linked to underactivity in the prefrontal cortex in the brain (Amen 2002 & 1999; Gray & Amen 2003; Volkow, Wang & Kollins, 2009).

The prefrontal cortex is located in the front of the brain, underneath the forehead.

Psychologist Vincent Monastra (2005), in his book, *Parenting Children With ADHD*, suggests that underactivity in the prefrontal cortex makes it difficult to think, plan, concentrate, and stay on task. With ADHD, the prefrontal cortex is not as active as it needs to be in order to succeed at school, work, and home.

Low activity in prefrontal cortex also equals low arousal. In other words, you just don't have enough juice to focus, pay attention, and get your work done. You find yourself distracted, thinking about other things, losing interest in the task at hand, and putting things off. Anything that's boring or monotonous causes you to shut down and tune out.

Juice Machines Inside Your Brain

Interestingly, the brain cells beneath the cortex (called subcortial nuclei) are sometimes called the "juice machines" (Mahoney & Restak, 1998). These brain cells give you enthusiasm and get-up-and-go energy. When these brain cells aren't stimulated or aroused, you'll find yourself feeling lethargic, sleepy, unmotivated, or bored.

A Closer Look at the Prefrontal Cortex Of The Brain

Let's take a look at the functions of the prefrontal cortex of the brain, as well as the problems that occur when the prefrontal cortex is underactive (or underaroused).

Functions Of The Prefrontal Cortex (Gray & Amen 2003):

- Attention span
- Perseverance
- Judgment
- Impulse control
- Organization
- Self-monitoring and supervision
- Problem solving
- Critical thinking
- Learning from experience
- Ability to feel and express emotions
- Interaction with the limbic system (amygdala & emotional gatekeeper of the brain)
- Empathy

Problems With The Prefrontal Cortex (Gray & Amen 2003):

- Short attention span
- Distractibility
- Impulse control
- Lack of perseverance
- Hyperactivity
- Chronic lateness, poor time management
- Disorganization
- Procrastination
- Unavailability of emotions
- Misperceptions
- Poor judgment
- Trouble learning from experience
- Short term memory problems
- Social and test anxiety

Boredom Causes Us To Tune Out

Gray & Amen (2003) contend that low dopamine and an underactive prefrontal cortex causes us to be bored. To stay on task, a task needs to be stimulating and arousing. Boredom causes us to tune out, like a computer monitor that fades to black, due to inactivity.

Stimulating Activities Turn On Our Brainpower

With children, ADHD disappears when they're playing video games. That's because it's a highly stimulating and arousing activity. ADHD adults are the same way. We seek immediate gratification, and we lose interest if we don't get it. Whenever we're required to do something that doesn't seem relevant or to the point, our brains begin to shut down.

A lack of stimulation is taxing on the brain and depletes dopamine (Gray & Amen, 2003). A lack of dopamine causes us to feel bored, tired, restless, hyperactive, impulsive, and disruptive.

With increased dopamine, we experience a surge in clarity, pleasure, energy, and motivation. Dopamine enables our prefrontal cortex to become more active. A brain fog lifts, and we experience a renewed sense of meaning and purpose.

As mentioned earlier, brain training with the ALERT will naturally boost your dopamine levels using the Sensory Motor Rhythm. The gentle rhythmic stimulation provokes your brain cells to wire and fire correctly, produce a stable supply of neurotransmitters, and successfully connect to neighboring neurons at the synapse. The ALERT also increases oxygen and blood flow to the brain. The ALERT does this with gentle light and sound stimulation to the visual cortex and auditory cortex. As a result, your brain naturally compensates for any neurotransmitter deficiency that it may be experiencing due to ADHD.

Natural Ways To Boost Neurotransmitter Levels

To produce dopamine, your body needs nourishment provided by amino acids. Even if you have an adequate supply of dopamine, your brain must be able to process it. Proper nutrition and exercise enables your brain to create and use dopamine, serotonin and other neurotransmitters. A lack of exercise and nutritional deficiencies can quickly cause an imbalance in brain chemistry. However, eating amino acid rich foods helps us to correct brain chemistry. The practical application of this research is called Activated Amino Acid Supplementation.

Practical Nutritional Tips For ADHD

Gray & Amen (2003) offers these practical nutritional tips for ADHD:

• The brain produces the next day's supply of dopamine from 10 pm to midnight, so it's wise to get to sleep early (p. 27).

• Make your diet high in protein, low in carbohydrates, low in fat, and eliminate simple sugars and carbohydrates. Refined carbohydrates have a negative impact on dopamine levels in the brain (p. 148).

• To produce more dopamine, avoid high glycemic foods. They lower the production of brain chemicals and create a serotonin spike which lowers dopamine levels (p. 257).

• For breakfast, enjoy a nutrient-dense breakfast shake that contains protein powder, flax seed, digestive enzymes, vitamins, ionic plant source minerals, water, and ice (p. 201-214). Or try a nutritional shake mix which contains natural amino acids. This can replace breakfast or supplement a light, healthful breakfast. For best results, repeat the shake in the evening, since dopamine is produced from 10 pm to midnight.

• Eat dopamine-producing foods. The top 20 are egg whites, whey, adzuki/ kidney/ lima/ mung beans, crab, cod, flounder, skim milk, abalone, lobster, clams, black beans, low fat cottage cheese, shrimp, sea bass, turkey, halibut, spirulina, chicken, refried beans, and wheat berry English muffins (p. 257-260).

• In addition to amino acids provided by proteins (for amino acid supplements,) you need healthy fats for the production of dopamine such as Omega 3 Fatty Acids found in: Flax seed; avocado; walnuts; fish such as tuna, salmon, mackerel, cod; pumpkin seeds; soybeans; kidney beans; flax seed oil; cod liver oil; hemp seed; hemp seed oil; and sea vegetables such as nori, hijiki, and kombu (p. 260-261).

• Cleanse your liver so it can function properly and produce and process amino acids which make dopamine. Enjoy a morning cleansing drink containing trace minerals, Aloe Vera, lemon juice, and honey. Or try Isagenix brand Fast Start Drink mix, which contains 70 organic plant source trace minerals and pure Aloe Vera juice. If you strengthen your digestion with digestive enzyme supplements and drink minerals and Aloe Vera to cleanse the liver, your body will more effectively digest proteins and fats to that the liver can process and convert amino acids into healthy brain chemistry (p. 21).

• Research demonstrates that various amino acid supplements increase dopamine and blood flow to the brain, such as tyrosine, grape seed or pine bark capsules, and ginkgo biloba. (p. 148- 149).

• Regular exercise reduces dopamine deficiency of ADD and ADHD (p. 98). It is generally recommended that you exercise 2 – 4 times a week, for 20 minutes or more.

"Until recently, the idea that food might profoundly and rapidly influence brain chemistry was considered scientifically ludicrous. Scientists thought the brain, of all organs, was particularly protected from the random permutations of nutrient invasions. It turns out that the brain is uniquely responsive to food chemicals... The radical conclusion: The type of neurotransmitters your neurons make and release and their ultimate destiny within the brain depend greatly on what you eat. Obviously, this makes food a very big regulator of the brain," writes Jean Carper (2000), in her book *Your Miracle Brain* (p. 9).

Dear Reader,

Have you ever had a lousy phone connection? It's frustrating! Sometimes, you can barely hear the person on the other end. You might yell, "Speak up!" or press the volume button. What's the problem? Perhaps there is a weak signal in the phone line.

It's the same thing with ADHD. Your brain is like a complex system of telephone wires. If a wire is broken or weak, then the communication signals shortcircuits, and stops dead in its tracks. The message doesn't go through, and power is lost. When this happens repeatedly, it results in an electro-chemical balance of the brain. This imbalance causes you to be distracted and disorganized.

The telephone helps people to talk to each other. In the same way, your brain cells (or neurons) have a system for talking to each other. There are about 50 miles of neurons running through your body, like a network of telephone wires.

Neurons relay messages between your brain, spinal chord, and body. These messages are in the form of tiny electro-chemical signals.

(Continued)

A brain cell consists of three parts: A cell body, dendrites, and an axon. Neurons look like trees, with offshoots of bushy branches called dendrites. Your dendrites act as antennas—transmitting and picking up signals from your brain cells. When brain cells talk to each other, at least five important things occur:

1. Your dendrites become thicker and denser.

2. Neurotransmitters are exchanged, so the "phone call" goes through.

3. The synapse (or space between brain cells) becomes stronger, which results in more durable neural connections.

4. Strong neural connections =
Better communication in the brain.

5. Improved thinking, concentration, focus, learning, and retention.

Bottom line: When you use the ALERT, the audio-visual stimulation encourages your brain cells to talk to each other, so that your telephone call goes through.

All the best,
Nicky

CHAPTER 8

ADHD & Increasing Electro-Chemical Communication Between Brain Cells

"Some of the most thrilling discoveries of how the brain works comes from the knowledge of neurotransmitter systems. It is these brain chemicals that substanctially define who you are, at every microsecond of your life. Flashing through neurons one by one, neurotransmitters lay down biochemical highways that carry your every thought and feeling through the brain's vast neuronal network. Without neurotransmitters, the lights in the brain would go out."— Jean Carper (2000), *Your Miracle Brain*, p. 8.

From an electro-chemical perspective, ADHD can be explained as wiring and firing problems in your brain. Your brain cells (neurons) are struggling to talk to each other, and make a connection. It's like talking on the phone when the sound is going in and out. In this chapter, we'll explore the concept of electro-chemical communication in the brain, and why it's important for your brain cells to talk to each other.

Hello, Is Anyone There?

Suppose you're talking on the phone, and can barely hear the person on the other end. You speak louder and louder, but it doesn't make any difference. You glance at the keypad, and push the volume button. Nothing seems to help. What's the use? You can't talk like this, or carry on a conversation. You can barely hear what the other person is saying. Perhaps there is a weak signal in the phone line.

It's the same thing that happens with ADHD. Your brain cells struggle to talk to each other, and make a connection. The problem is that your brain cells tend to misfire and miswire, or there aren't enough neurotransmitters for the signal to go through.

Your brain is like a complex system of wires. If a wire is broken or weak, then communication signals don't go through. When a signal short circuits, it stops dead in its tracks. The message doesn't go through, and power is lost. When this happens repeatedly, it results in an electro-chemical balance of the brain. This imbalance causes you to be distracted and disorganized. Researchers suggest that memory is destroyed through a disruption of neurotransmitters (Gottlieb, 2001; Volkow, Wang & Fowler, 2001; Volkow, Wang & Kollins, 2009; Carper, 2000; & Sprenger, 1999). It is critical that you have sufficient amounts of neurotransmitters in order for your brain to be chemically balanced.

"How well a brain conducts electro-chemical business between cells appears more crucial to memory, intelligence, and mood than the total number of neurons tucked under the skull. What really matters is not the size of your brain, or how many neurons are left, but how it is wired, and what you can do to preserve or rejuvenate the wiring, if necessary," says Jean Carper (2000) in *Your Miracle Brain*, p. 14.

Let's go back to the telephone. You decide to call your friend back. You pick up the receiver, but there is no dial tone. Why isn't the phone working? Perhaps the phone line is down. There could be a loose connection somewhere within the phone itself. Maybe the wires are broken or frayed. Or maybe the plug in the wall is loose, and there is no electrical power going to the receiver. What if the circuit breaker is not properly connected? If that's the case, the power isn't even getting into the house. Hmm, there are many possibilities why the phone isn't working. There could be electrical disconnections in any number of places.

It is frustrating when your phone doesn't work properly. After all, you're trying to call someone who is important to you. You have a lot on your mind, and are eager to talk to them. If only this telephone would work properly... then you could call them up and make plans. If only, if only, if only...

How Your Brain Works

Your brain is an electro-chemical communication network. It is similar to a telephone, in that your brain cells need to talk to each other. Your brain uses tiny electrical signals to help you to see, hear, taste, smell, and touch.

All of this sensory input is driven by electrical signals than run through your nerves to your brain. Let's break down the process a little more.

The brain consists of billions of tiny cells called neurons. Each neuron maintains itself in an electrically-charged state. It receives electrical signals from other neurons, and passes them on to others. What actually happens is that a tiny amount of neurotransmitters (brain chemicals) are released from the terminals of the neuron. This chemical excites an electrical response in the neuron that is next in the chain, and so the signal moves onward.

In the case of ADHD, there isn't enough of the neurotransmitter dopamine to excite neurons that are involved in reasoning and attention. Reasoning involves the inhibition of emotion and impulsiveness. When your brain excites the "reasoning" neurons, you inhibit emotion and impulsiveness. A deficiency of dopamine results in ADHD symptoms.

All the functions of the brain (including feeling, seeing, thinking, and moving muscles) depend on electrical signals being passed from one neuron to the next. The normal brain is constantly generating electrical rhythms in this way. The constant buzz of electro-chemical signals in our bodies is what enables us to think, feel, and respond.

A Network Of Telephone Wires

The telephone helps people to talk to each other. In the same way, your brain cells (or neurons) have a system for talking to each other. When your brain cells talk to each other, memory and learning occurs. There are about 50 miles of neurons running through your body, like a network of telephone wires (Parker, 1999). Neurons relay messages between your brain, spinal chord, and body. These messages are in the form of tiny electro-chemical signals.

Three Parts Of A Neuron

A neuron consists of three parts:
(1) Cell body
(2) Dendrites
(3) Axon

As you can see from Illustration 8:1 below, neurons look like trees, with offshoots of bushy branches called dendrites. Your dendrites act as antennas—transmitting and picking up signals from your brain cells. Healthy dendrites are thick and dense. The thicker and denser your dendrites, the better you are able to think and remember.

(Illustration 8:1) A neuron consists of three parts.

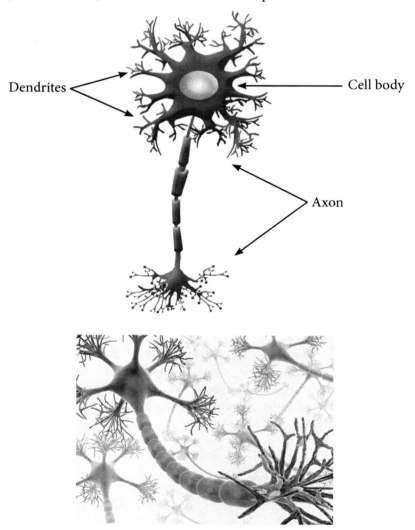

(Illustration 8:2) Electrical signals travel down the axon to the dendrites.

The long, thin, cord-like extension from the cell body is called the axon. The axon acts like a telephone wire carrying messages from the neuron. The message starts with an electrical signal in the cell body, going down the axon to the dendrites (Illustration 8:2). Once the electrical signal reaches the tip of the dendrites, there is a little round bulb—which is a storage sack for neurotransmitters. In order for your brain cells to talk to each other, there must be enough neurotransmitters for the electrical signal to be picked up by the neighboring neuron (Illustration 8:3).

Here's the challenge: There is a gap between brain cells. For your brain cells to talk to each other, the electrical signal must be strong enough to cross the gap and spark interest in the receiving cell. There must be enough neurotransmitters for the electrical signal to flash across the gap, and make a connection (Illustration 8:4).

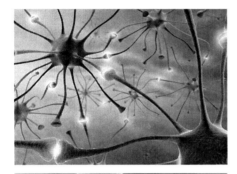

(Illustration 8:3)
Neurons firing and wiring neurotransmitters.

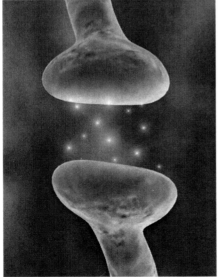

(Illustration 8:4)
Close-up of the gap between brain cells. In order for your brain cells to talk to each other, the electrical signal must cross the gap and spark interest in the receiving cell.

Neurotransmitters Are Gatekeepers

Neurotransmitters are gatekeepers. They control whether or not the brain cells fire and wire. When electrical signals are present on an axon, it's the neurotransmitters that determine whether it will cross the synapse into the next dendrite. Excitatory neurotransmitters such as dopamine can help a weak signal appear strong to the next neuron. Addictions largely increase dopamine, so the effect is very strong and the addiction is tough to rehabilitate from. Neurotransmitters such as GABA and serotonin largely have an inhibitory effect and will calm an agitated brain down. Basic nutrition such as minerals (zinc, selenium, magnesium) and other nutrients such as tryptophan, vitamin B, vitamin D and omega 3s, also help to regulate brain function.

Another thing that boosts neurotransmitters is stimulation. When you stimulate and arouse your brain, you will experience a boost in your neurotransmitter levels. This is exactly what the ALERT does. The ALERT provides your brain with audio-visual stimulation that encourages your brain cells to exchange neurotransmitters, so that they can fire and wire together. The end result is that you brain cells talk to each other. When this happens, your ADHD symptoms fade away.

It's An Electro-Chemical Process

Neurotransmitters are chemicals that carry information from one brain cell (or neuron) to another. The process is electro-chemical. The activity within the neuron itself is electrical, and the interaction with other neurons is chemical.

An electrical impulse causes the neuron to release neurotransmitters, which swim across the gap called the synapse. The synapse is the small space between neurons, and neurotransmitters attach themselves to the dendrite of the receiving neuron. Next, the chemical message in the synapse is converted into an electrical message. This enables the brain cell to generate an action potential, which is actually an electrical current. That electrical current goes down the axon to the next neuron in the chain. This process repeats itself over and over, as your brain cells talk to each other.

Your Brain Cells Talking To Each Other = Learning

Neuroscientists define learning as two neurons talking to each other (Kandel, 2007). This process that you've just read about is how your brain cells learn. When one neuron sends a message to another neuron, neurotransmitters are exchanged, and communication (talking) and learning take place. With this happens repeatedly, the connection between neurons becomes stronger. The gaps between neurons become stronger. As the neurons repeatedly fire (or talk to each other) the dendrites and axons get used to these connections. With each connection, the transmission of brain cells becomes faster and easier.

New Experiences Makes Your Synapses Multiply

Your synapses (or connections between neurons) multiply in response to new experiences (Mahoney & Restak, 1998; Hawley, 2000; Kandel, 2007). Learning occurs when fresh synapses sprout, or when existing connections are modified in response to new information. Your brain creates new brain cell synapses (connections) and prunes old ones in response to experience. Your brain is plastic (or changeable) and grows new pathways and connections in response to changes in its environment. This goes on throughout life.

Path In The Woods

The way your brain cells talk and learn is similar to a path in the woods (Sprenger, 1999). The first time you walk in the woods, there may not be a path. The grass and weeds are rough and overgrown. With each step, you push the grass and weeds beneath your feet. Stray branches and weeds may even poke or brush against you. The next time you go into the woods, it is easier because you have previously walked over the weeds. There aren't as many obstacles in your path. Each time you walk in the woods, the path becomes smoother and more defined. In the same way, your brain cells (neurons) become more and more efficient with each connection. Stronger connections mean that information travels faster. In other words, you can think and act faster because your brain is wiring and firing, and the connections are getting stronger each time. With each connection, you are reinforcing and solidifying the neural pathways in the brain. Eventually, this process (electro-chemical communication in the brain) becomes very automatic and comfortable, like an path in the woods that is often traveled.

Brain Cells That Fire Together, Wire Together

It is known as Hebb's Law: "Neurons (or brain cells) that fire together, wire together" (Hebb, 1949). In other words, your brain cells must fire enough neurotransmitters across the gap in order to wire together. If the connection is successful, then your brain cells are talking to each other and learning. It is called synaptic transmission, and it happens very fast—in milliseconds.

The brain's electro-chemical signals are fast, all-or-nothing, nerve impulses. When your brain's signals connect successfully, then communication, learning, and memory take place. If the brain's signal connection fizzles out, and stops dead in its tracks, then there isn't a complete response from the brain. There is a breakdown in communication, learning, and memory.

The brain uses the electro-chemical signals to receive, analyze, and convey information. The brain analyzes and interprets patterns of incoming electro-chemical signals—and uses these signals to create our every day sensations of sight, touch, taste, smell, and sound.

Five Things That Happen When Brain Cells Talk To Each Other:

1. **Dendrites become thicker and denser.** As your brain cells repeatedly talk to each other, the dendrites and axons are strengthening their connections. They become thicker and denser. The next time your brain cells try to talk to each other, the connection is easier to make.

2. **Neurotransmitters are exchanged**, so the "phone call" goes through.

3. **Strength in the gap.** The synapse (or gap between brain cells) becomes stronger as your brain cells talk to each other. This results in stronger and more durable neural connections.

4. **Stronger neural connections = better communication in the brain.** The more your brain cells talk to each other (and learn) the faster and stronger the neural connections become. The more your brain accesses its neural pathways, the stronger and more defined they become.

Stronger connections means that information travels faster. In other words, you can think and act faster because your brain is wiring and firing, and the connections are getting stronger each time. With each connection, you are reinforcing and solidifying the neural pathways in the brain.

5. **Improved thinking, concentration, focus, learning, and retention.** As your brain cells become more efficient at connecting and talking to each other, your mental processing speed increases. Your ability to think, focus, concentrate, and learn improves (Mahoney & Restak, 1998; Sprenger, 1999; Kandel, Schwartz & Jessell, 2000).

ADHD & Neurotransmitter Problems

With ADHD, there is a disruption in the normal order of your brain cells talking to each other and exchanging neurotransmitters. It could be one of two problems: (1) deficiency, or not enough neurotransmitters or (2) disruption, or unstable connections between brain cells. Both of these problems short circuit the communication inside your brain, and cause you to be distracted and disorganized (Mahoney & Restak, 1998; Carper, 2000).

Neurotransmitter Deficiency

With ADHD, there may not be enough neurotransmitters for brain cells to make a connection. As a result, the communication between brain cells is weak or ineffective. When there aren't enough active neurotransmitters (dopamine) then you can't stimulate a complete response from the brain.

Neurotransmitters are important brain chemicals. As mentioned before, neurotransmitters carry your thoughts and feelings from one brain cell to the next. They are the essence of focus, concentration, memory, and creativity.

If you've felt euphoric because of something wonderful that has happened to you, then you know firsthand what neurotransmitters are. They are the "feel-good" brain chemicals that make you feel happy and excited. They also create arousal, which enables you to focus and pay attention. Neurotransmitters enable us to lose ourselves in physical exercise, or some other activity that you're extremely passionate about, like video games or maybe shopping. If you don't have enough neurotransmitters, it is difficult to stay on-track and concentrate.

Disruption Or Unstable Connections Between Brain Cells

With ADHD, your brain cells might also be misfiring or miswiring. If neurotransmitters misfire, then the signal does not go through. As a result, there isn't a complete response from the brain. The neural connections in your brain gradually become unstable, and create interference. It's like hearing static on the phone. Most people respond by hanging up. The sound is so distorted that you can't clearly hear the person on the other end. When unstable connections occur between brain cells, it creates dysfunctional pathways in the brain. The more you think and behave in this way, the more reinforced this path becomes. After a while, the ADHD response is automatic. In other words, you will automatically experience distraction, poor focus and concentration, restlessness, impulsiveness, and disorganization. You will naturally think and act according to these ingrained neural pathways. After a while, your brain interprets ADHD as normal.

Don't Settle For A Lousy Phone Connection!

Having ADHD is like a phone that isn't reliable. You aren't able to con-centrate, focus, and get things done—and it might be because of small, gradual glitches in your brain cells. When these glitches go unrepaired, it leads to screw-ups in the brain's circuitry. Eventually, your brain cells lose their capacity to send and receive messages. There just isn't enough power for the call to go through.

With ADHD, your brain's biochemical activities are in disharmony. This disharmony makes it difficult to concentrate, focus, and remember.

What's the solution? Tune up the electro-chemical communication in your brain. In other words, train your brain to restore its electro-chemical balance, so that the telephone call can go through.

When you get your phone fixed, your brain cells will talk to each other. But, who will fix your phone line? It's not your doctor or pharmacist. You don't need Ritalin to fix this problem. Instead, you need to stimulate and activate your brain using your brain's natural electricity. Like jumper cables on a dead car battery, you need a jump-start.

With the ALERT, you will ramp up your brain's natural electricity, and condition your brain for peak performance. You can restore the electro-chemical communication inside your brain. You will train your brain cells to wire and fire correctly, produce a stable supply of neurotransmitters, and successfully connect to neighboring neurons at the synapse. With the ALERT, your brain is stimulated and activated with the Rhythm of Peak Performance, or Sensory Motor Rhythm. By correcting the electro-chemical imbalances of ADHD, you will experience dramatic improvements in concentration, memory, coping skills, and more.

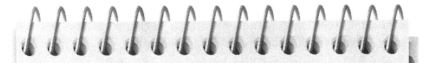

Dear Reader,

The rhythmic activity of your brain is expressed as brainwaves. On paper, your brainwaves look like wavy lines. Brainwave frequencies are described in terms of hertz (Hz) or cycles per second (cps), which are measured by an EEG (or electroencephalogram).

There are four types of brainwaves: Beta, alpha, theta and delta. You're always in one of these brainwave states, or a combination of them.

The Sensory Motor Rhythm is a type of beta brainwave which has been scientifically proven to be ideal for reading, writing, studying, or task completion. It is used in the ALERT program to interrupt your ADHD, and reprogram your brain for peak performance.

In your brain, there is a dominant brainwave frequency, or place where you're "parked." The problem with ADHD is that you're parked in the wrong place. You're in the wrong place at the wrong time. Because you're parked in the wrong place, you'll tend to be distracted, impulsive, and thrill-seeking—when you're supposed to be paying attention and concentrating.

(Continued)

Because you're parked in the wrong place, your brain interprets ADHD as normal, and works to maintain it. Unfortunately, your brainwaves will not return to a healthy balance on their own. Your brain will continue to function that way, unless you do something about it.

Have you ever watched TV, and the announcer says, "We interrupt this program to bring you a very special announcement?" This type of interruption is exactly what your brain needs in order to stop ADHD. In order to change, your ADHD brainwaves must be interrupted.

How can you interrupt your ADHD? With the ALERT, of course. You can interrupt your ADHD brainwaves with the sights and sounds of the ALERT. It gently nudges your brain with the Rhythm of Peak Performance. This rhythm stimulates and arouses the brain, and nudges it in the direction of a healthier balance.

When you train your brainwaves with the ALERT, you're stimulating and balancing your brainwaves, so that they will operate at peak capacity, and work to create equilibrium in your body. By taming your brainwaves, you can conquer ADHD.

All the best,
Nicky

CHAPTER 9

Understanding Your Brainwaves

"How do you know that you have brainwaves? You cannot directly feel them. The only reason you know that you have brainwaves is because you've been told that you do. Of course, we could measure them, if we had the right equipment, but few of us will have the experience of seeing our brain as it is observed through advanced scientific equipment. In fact, even in that case, the scientist is not seeing the brainwaves themselves. These waves are invisible to all the senses. They can be translated into a measurable form only through scientific technology. Does this means that you have to seek out a scientific laboratory or buy some expensive equipment to check on the health of your brainwaves? Not at all. The evidence of your brainwaves is all around you. It is evident in the quality of the relationships you have, in the emotions you carry, and in the choices you make. Everything in your life is the direct result of your brainwaves." —Ilchi Lee (2008), *Brainwave Vibration: Getting Back Into The Rhythm Of A Happy, Healthy Life.*

Suppose you asked someone on the street, "What are brainwaves?" They would probably shrug their shoulders, and admit, "I dunno!" Or maybe they'll tell you that brainwaves come from the brain. Of course, this is a very limited understanding. We may not realize it, but our brainwaves are a driving force in our lives. Our brainwaves affect everything we think, say, and do.

Many books and articles have been written about brainwaves. Much of this material is complicated and difficult to understand. That is why I've written this chapter, to give you basic understanding about brainwaves.

As you know, I'm not a medical doctor with a history of working with patients. I'm not a Ph.D. researcher who has spent my life conducting experiments in various laboratories. However, I'll share with you information that I've discovered by reading books and articles, and talking to experts in the field.

I've spent three years writing and researching this book. Understanding ADHD and how the brain works has become an obsession for me. I've spent a lot of time and energy trying to making sense of all this. Much of my research was frustrating, because the literature was long-winded and hard to understand. You know, the type of book or article that makes you shake your head, and wonder, "What in the world are they trying to say?" And, "Why are they making this so complicated? Come on, let's get to the point!" Or worse, books that are so boring that you have to slap yourself to pay attention. If you have ADHD, you know exactly what I mean. Boring is like a ticket to hell. Your eyes glaze over and zone out. Your brain shuts down, like the screen saver on your computer when there is no activity. If nothing else, I'd like to spare you from that incredibly frustrating experience.

Perhaps that is what I bring to the table. I wanted to make this book easy to understand, and interesting to read. I wanted to spare you the hassle of plowing through the literature and trying to figure things out on your own. By reading this book, you will quickly grasp what's taken me a long time to figure out. You're also in an excellent position to take things to the next level. If you wanted to, you could read other books about brainpower and ADHD, and continue to learn more about this fascinating subject.

This chapter will give you a basic understanding of brainwaves. You will learn about the four types of brainwaves, and why brainwaves are important to ADHD. By the time you finish reading this chapter, you will know more about brainwaves than the average person on the street. You don't have to be an expert, but you'll know enough to make the most of your ALERT brain training.

What Are Brainwaves?

Your brain is made up of billions of neurons which use electricity and chemicals to talk to each other and learn. The combined electrical activity (billions of brain cells talking and sending electrical signals) is called a "brainwave pattern."

Brainwaves reflect the rhythmic activity of the brain. On paper, brainwaves look like wavy lines because of their cyclic, wave-like nature.

Brainwave frequencies are described in terms of hertz (Hz) or cycles per second (cps), which are measured by an EEG (or electroencephalogram).

Four Types Of Brainwaves

There are four types of brainwaves: Delta, theta, alpha and beta. Let's take a closer look at each of these.

Delta (0.1 to 4 Hz): When you're sleeping deeply (but not dreaming), you tend to be in a delta brainwave state. In delta, your brainwaves are of the greatest amplitude and slowest frequency. They typically range from 1 to 4 cycles per second. They never go down to zero because that would indicate the absence of brainwaves, or clinical death. However, deep and dreamless sleep will take you down to the lowest frequency, which is 2 to 3 cycles a second.

Theta (4 to 8 Hz): Have you ever driven on the highway, and discovered that you can't remember the last five miles? This is an example of a theta brainwave state. You tend to disengage from the task at hand. You may daydream or reflect on other things. In theta, we also experience flashes of insight. We may have "eureka" or "light bulb" experiences. In this way, theta can be a very positive and creative mental state.

Alpha (8 to 13 Hz). In an alpha brainwave state, you're relaxed, but are aware of what is happening around you. Alpha represents a state of non-arousal. Alpha brainwaves are slower and higher in amplitude. You're probably in alpha when you're watching TV after a long hectic day.

Another time that you're probably in alpha is when you're relaxing deeply, meditating, praying, or taking a casual stroll in the yard. Alpha brainwave rhythms produce peaceful feelings, warm hands and feet, a sense of well-being, improved sleep, improved academic performance, increased productivity at work, reduced anxiety, and improved immunity.

Beta (12 to 35 Hz). Beta brainwaves range from relaxed thought to being awake and focused. If you're strongly engaged in writing or reading, then you're probably in a beta state. The frequency of beta waves cover a wide range: Low, medium and high. Beta waves are present in a strongly engaged mind. You're probably in beta when you're talking or having a conversation. You might even be excitedly making a speech or teaching a class while in a beta brainwave state.

Three Types Of Beta Brainwaves:

Low beta (12 to 15 Hz) = Relaxed or passive attention.
Mid beta (15 to 20 Hz) = Active attention.
High beta (21 to 35 Hz) = Anxious attention.

Later, we will discuss the Sensory Motor Rhythm which is a type of low beta brainwave which has been scientifically proven to be ideal for reading, writing, studying, or task completion. (This is the Rhythm of Peak Performance that was mentioned in the previous chapters). Low beta involves relaxed thinking. Mid beta involves active attention. High beta occurs when you're anxious and struggling with restless energy.

Different Types Of Brainwaves (Illustration 9:1)

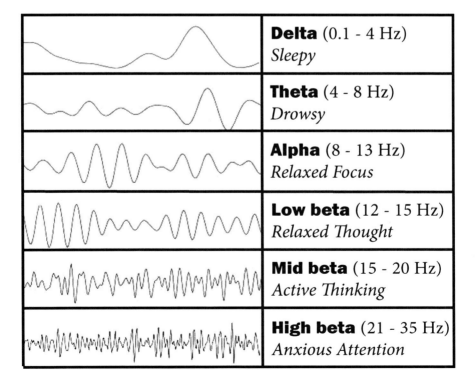

	Delta (0.1 - 4 Hz) *Sleepy*
	Theta (4 - 8 Hz) *Drowsy*
	Alpha (8 - 13 Hz) *Relaxed Focus*
	Low beta (12 - 15 Hz) *Relaxed Thought*
	Mid beta (15 - 20 Hz) *Active Thinking*
	High beta (21 - 35 Hz) *Anxious Attention*

Throughout the day, we constantly transition from one brainwave state to another brainwave state. Let's take a look at some of these transitions.

Quick Transitions Between Brainwave States

Fast asleep in your bed	To waking up and getting up.
Going about your day, thinking about "whatever"	To focusing on a specific task or assignment that requires your time, attention and concentration.
You're driving the car on your way home, and feel casually relaxed, easy going, no worries	Another driver had an accident, and you must pay careful attention to ensure your safety. Suddenly, you're in a state of persistent, heightened alert.
Being by yourself	To being with another person, a group of people, or in a crowd.
Walking down the hallway	To sitting down and reading, writing or listening to a speaker.
Warm-up stretches	To fast-paced physical exercise.
Fast-paced physical exercise, you're sweaty and slightly out of breath	To being in a state of flow, where you gain momentum, and the exercise seems easy and effortless.
Casually reading, thinking, and reflecting	To a eureka moment, "aha" or light bulb experience which gives you an incredible flash of insight.
Wide awake, many thoughts racing through your head	To settling down, reading a book, watching TV, getting ready for bed, or going to sleep.

Your Brain's Electrical Profile Constantly Changes

All of these situations involve a quick transition between brainwave states. With each mental state, the electrical profile of your brain changes. Your brain cells must quickly transition from one state to the next. You definitely don't want to get stuck in the wrong brainwave state. When that happens, you may find yourself performing like a run down car—stalling, idling, unable to shift gears, or shutting down completely.

Brainwaves Cause And Correct Problems

Did you know that your brainwaves can cause problems… and also correct problems? For instance, if you're struggling to get up in the morning, your theta brainwaves may be to blame. You may have too much theta brainwaves. This causes you to be drowsy, lethargic, and stuck in sleep mode.

Suppose you get up anyway, and go to work or school. You still feel sluggish. Once you arrive, you try to read a book. You just can't seem to focus your eyes on the text, and understand the words on the page. You stop and start over. What's the problem? It may be a lack of alpha brainwaves.

Your Brain Cells Must Go In And Out Of Park Quickly

Alpha brainwaves are considered a parking and resting condition for the neurons of the brain (Swingle, 2008). It is like driving a car, and shifting gears to go forward or backward. In the same way, your brain cells must go in and out of park quickly. As you open and close your eyes, your brain must make a quick transition from rest to being ready for activity.

Insomnia: Stuck In The Wrong Brainwave State

Have you ever been so wound up that you're unable to fall asleep? This is another example of being stuck in the wrong brainwave state. When this happens, you're probably stuck in high beta brainwaves. What you need to do is transition to delta brainwaves, which help you to sleep. Easier said than done, right? Well, you can interupt your brainwaves by getting out of bed, and making yourself a cup of herbal tea. Perhaps you have other ways for dealing with insomnia, but the point is that you need to transition to another brainwave state, so that you can get some rest.

ADHD: Parked In The Wrong Place

With ADHD, your brainwaves are parked in the wrong place, at the wrong time. You might be parked in a low arousal brainwave state, when you really need to be in a "let's get busy" state. When you're bored—which neuroscientists say is low arousal—the chances that you'll be productive are slim to none. The trick is to gradually boost the speed of your brainwaves, so you can transition to a state of mind that enables you to concentrate, focus, and get things done.

Cycling Through The Brainwave States

When you go to sleep at night, your brainwaves cycles through all four stages: Beta, alpha, theta and delta. For instance, when you settle down in bed and read for a few minutes, you are likely to be in low beta. If you watch TV, you're likely to be in alpha. If you put your book down, turn off the lights, and close your eyes, your brainwaves will descend from beta, to alpha, to theta, and finally, when you fall asleep, to delta.

What happens to your brainwaves when you dream? Active dreaming takes place when your delta brainwave frequencies increase into the frequency of theta brainwaves. This is when Rapid Eye Movement (or REM) occurs. Your eyes actually move fast and pulse when you're dreaming.

Suppose you've slept all night, and now it is morning. Your alarm clock goes off. Beep, beep, beep! As you wake up, your brainwave frequencies will cycle through the four stages of brainwave activity. As you slowly awaken, your brainwaves increase from delta to theta. You may remember some of your dreams. You still feel sleepy, but you need to get up. You might put on some music, or turn on your TV. As you listen to the music or watch the news, your brainwaves gradually cycle into an alpha state. As you gradually begin to focus on the day ahead of you, your brainwaves cycle into beta.

To recap, there are four brainwave states that range from deep dreamless sleep (theta) to high arousal (high beta). These brainwaves occur in women, men, and children. They are consistent across cultures and countries. Everyone has brainwaves, and they affect everything that you think, say, and do.

Seven Things To Keep In Mind About Brainwaves

Here are seven things to keep in mind about brainwaves, as they relate to ADHD:

1. **The rhythmic activity of your brain is expressed as brainwaves.** In other words, you're in a beta, alpha, theta, or delta brainwave state—or a combination of these brainwave frequencies.

2. **Your dominant brainwave is where you're parked.** Your brain produces various brainwaves, but there is always a single brainwave or band that is higher than others. That brainwave (or band of brainwaves) will be dominant. Of course, the other brainwaves are present in trace amounts at all times. In other words, a person giving a debate is in high beta, but their brainwaves have traces of alpha, theta and delta. When you're in a predominant brainwave state, neuroscientists say that you're "parked" there.

3. **With ADHD, you're parked in the wrong place.** You're in the wrong place at the wrong time. Because you're parked in the wrong place, you'll tend to be distracted, impulsive, and thrill-seeking—when you're supposed to be paying attention and concentrating. Your brainwaves always correspond to your mental state.

4. **Because you're parked in the wrong place, your brainwaves don't fit the task at hand.** With ADHD, there is a mismatch between what you're doing and how your brain works. Suppose you need to write a report and turn it in. Ideally, you need to be in a beta brainwave state. If you're sleepy, and struggling to keep your eyes open, then you're in a theta brainwave state. In order to write your report, you'll need to transition to beta brainwaves—at least long enough to get your work done. Ideally, you want your brainwaves to fit the task at hand.

5. Your brain interprets ADHD as normal, and works to maintain it. Unfortunately, your brainwaves will not return to a healthy balance on their own. Your brain will continue to function that way, unless you do something about it. Your brain is stuck in an ADHD pattern.

6. In order to change, your ADHD brainwaves must be interrupted. With the sights and sounds of the ALERT, you can interrupt your ADHD brainwaves. You can gently nudge your brain with the Rhythm of Peak Performance. This rhythm stimulates and arouses the brain, and nudges it in the direction of a healthier balance.

7. In order to change, the tempo of your brainwaves needs to be stabilized. By using the ALERT brain training system, you finetune, balance, and stabilize your brainwaves. The trick is to adjust the speed of your brainwaves to a normal range, with smooth brainwave transitions between states. By taming your brainwaves, you can conquer ADHD.

Quality Of Your Brainwaves Affects The Quality Of Your Life

Healthy brainwaves equal a healthy body. Your brain is in constant communication with the parts of your body, various organs and bodily processes. When you train your brainwaves with the ALERT, you're stimulating and balancing your brainwaves, so that they operate at peak capacity, and work to create equilibrium in your body.

A Very Brief History Of The EEG

• The brain produces electrical signals called brainwaves. The recording of brainwaves is called an EEG, or electroencephalogram. Actually, the device used to record brainwaves is also called an EEG.

• An EEG measures and records the electrical activity of your brain. Special sensors (electrodes) are attached to your head and hooked by wires to a computer. The computer records your brain's electrical activity on the screen as wavy lines.

• The first EEG was made in 1924 by Hans Berger, German medical doctor.

• Ten years after the discovery of brainwaves, British electrophysiologists Adrian and Matthews (1934) confirmed Dr. Berger's basic observations. They also presented research that proved brainwaves could be changed with flashing lights (a case for audio-visual entrainment).

• The importance of Dr. Berger's discoveries in EEG were finally recognized at an international forum in 1937. By 1938, electroencephalography started to be used by hospitals and research facilities in the United States, England, and France. Today, the EEG continues to be used to measure brainwaves (Wiedemann, 1994).

Dear Reader,

Whatever you're going through, you need a specific level of arousal and awareness. It's all about brainwaves, or the rhythmic activity of the brain. The tempo needs to be just right. Not too much of certain brainwave, nor too little, but just right.

In this next chapter, you'll find a chart that lists the possible effects of brainwaves. When you have the right amount of a brainwave frequency, you have equilibrium. Too much of a brainwave frequency results in hyperactivity. Too little of a brainwave frequency results in sluggishness.

A healthy brain is able to change brainwave states quickly, and move to the appropriate level of awareness. In contrast, the ADHD brain is not processing information at the right speed. It is either too slow or too fast. For this reason, your brain is not communicating information correctly to itself, so it is out-of-sync with itself. This is why you're not ready to do things to the best of your ability.

The good news is that you don't have to park in the wrong place. With the ALERT, you can crank up your engine, shift gears, and back out of that parking spot. You can find a new place to park that is just right for you.

All the best,
Nicky

CHAPTER 10

Balancing The Tempo Of Your Brainwaves

"A peak performing brain can combine its instruments (delta, theta, alpha and beta brainwaves) to play any tune demanded by life, shift states as needed, and enhance the outcome of any situation." — Norris, S. & Currieri, M. (1999), *Journal of Genetic Psychology.*

Whatever you're doing, it's best that your brainwaves fit the task at hand. You need certain brainwaves to be dominant, depending upon the circumstances or situation. You also need the tempo of your brainwaves to be just right. You don't want too much of a certain brainwave nor too little. You need the tempo to be just right.

A healthy brain is able to change brainwave states quickly, and move to the appropriate level of awareness. In contrast, the ADHD brain is not processing information at the right speed. It is either too slow or too fast. For this reason, your brain is not communicating information correctly to itself, so it is out-of-sync with itself. This is why you're not ready to do things to the best of your ability.

Stimulating Various Brainwave States

When you use the ALERT, you are rhythmically coaxing the brain into various brainwave states. The light and sound stimulation acts as an entraining signal to stimulate and arouse your brainwaves, and gently nudge them in a healthy direction.

On the next page is a list of possible brainwave effects (adapted from Swingle, 2008 and Hill & Castro, 2002). Each brainwave frequency has an intended outcome, ideal, or just the right amount of brainwaves. There are also pitfalls, if there is too much (or too little) of a particular brainwave.

Possible Effects of Brainwaves

Name Of Brainwave	Just The Right Amount Of These Brainwaves (Equilibrium & balance)
Beta	When beta waves are their best, you will experience a strongly engaged mindset. You are able to focus, concenrate and remember. For instance, you might be strongly engaged in talking, listening, writing, reading. or doing an assignment.
Alpha	When alpha waves are at their best, you will feel calm and relaxed, but aware of what is happening around you. Alpha represents a state of non-arousal.
Theta	When theta waves are at their best, you will experience flashes of insight, eureka or "light bulb" experiences. Theta brainwaves help us to disengage from the task at hand, and begin to think deeply, reflect, imagine, fantasize or daydream.
Delta	When delta waves are at their best, you will experience deep and dreamless sleep.

Too Much
Of These Brainwaves
(High, fast, excessive, hyperactive)

Too Little
Of These Brainwaves
(Low, slow, deficient, or sluggish)

Too much beta:
- Anxiety & restless
- Nervous energy
- Impatient
- Jittery
- Frantic
- Mind chatter

Too little beta:
- Struggle to get organized
- Distracted
- All over-the-place

Too much alpha:
- Can't finish projects
- Holding on to negative emotions and the past
- Afraid to try new things
- "Looping"—going over the same things repeatedly
- Difficulty letting go & moving on
- Afraid to relax and let go
- Struggle to visualize, or develop mental pictures

Too little alpha:
- Bored
- Lethargic
- Can't seem to get motivated
- Overwhelmed
- Sluggish, apathetic
- No energy
- Depressed, sad, gloomy

Too much theta:
- Struggle to pay attention because your mind wanders
- Too much daydreaming, or can't seem to snap out of it.
- Trouble waking up or excessive drowsiness
- Absence of directed thought

Too little theta:
- Afraid to let guard down
- Struggle to wind down or relax
- Lack of creative ideas
- Struggle to imagine or develop mental pictures
- Low stress tolerance
- Predisposition to addiction

Too much delta:
- Mental fog or fatigue
- Pain

Too little delta:
- Poor sleep, wake up frequently, or feel exhausted upon waking

Benefits Of Stimulating Your Brainwaves

Let's take a closer look at the various brainwave states, and how stimulating your brainwaves can benefit you.

Beta: By stimulating beta, you develop the ability to think fast, generate new ideas, and be productive. This type of fast mental processing definitely helps with taking tests, doing math problems, giving presentations, or completing projects.

Did you know that beta brainwaves naturally increase when a person talks? If you're interested in becoming more social and outgoing, a boost of beta brainwaves might be exactly what you need. Beta brainwaves enable you to think fast on your feet, so you are able to take initiative. You can determine what needs to be done and do it. In most people, an increase in beta activity speeds up your reaction time, ability to focus, and mental alertness.

Beta brainwaves are also the perfect antidote for mental fog, poor focus, or distractibility. Ritalin (and other ADHD drugs) tend to increase the beta brainwave activity in the brain. However, the ALERT will enable you to get similar results by stimulating your brain with the Sensory Motor Rhythm. Stimulating beta brainwaves is also useful for lifting depression and anxiety. Beta brainwaves also enhance your ability to write and think creatively.

Alpha: By stimulating alpha, you can reduce stress, anxiety, and feelings of paranoia. Typically, alpha brainwaves induce relaxation and calmness. As you relax into an alpha state, you will release muscle tension from the body, and lower your blood pressure. A boost of alpha brainwaves can help to curb and eliminate addictions.

Theta: By stimulating theta brainwaves, you will find yourself deeply relaxed. However, there is much more to theta than just relaxation. It is also a brainwave state where healing, restoration, and rejuvenation take place.

In a theta state, your brain produces many beneficial neuronicchemicals, such as acetylcholine, catecholamines, and vasopressin (Kandel, Schwartz

& Jessell, 2000). Researchers have found that acetylcholine is vital for long term memory. When acetylcholine production in the brain is high, we experience a boost in our long-term memory (Hasselmoa, 2006).

Interestingly, people with lower levels of acetylcholine tend to struggle with tasks involving learning and memory. Lower levels of acetylcholine also results in low arousal, or not being able to can't get into gear. This is not your imagination, nor is it laziness or apathy. There are certain chemicals that your brain needs to focus, concentrate, and remember. When you don't have enough of them, you will experience low arousal. This makes it difficult to get organized, focus, plan, or simply stay on task until your work is finished.

When you stimulate your theta brainwaves, your brain produces a stable supply of neurotransmitters, which enables you to learn and memorize more effectively. When you stimulate your brainwaves with the ALERT, your brain naturally produces the brain chemicals that you need to learn, remember, and think fast on your feet.

It seems counter-intuitive that deep relaxation would speed up your reaction time. In our society, we tend to think that a high pressure situation is exactly what we need to get our act together. Sure, some stress is good, but too much pressure can quickly become overwhelming. Too much stress causes us to feel emotionally drained, overwhelmed, frustrated, and helpless. In this state, it is really hard to come up with new ideas, take a fresh approach or try something new. What's the solution? Try a quick theta boost (a nap, a 22-minute ALERT session, taking a break, etc). to relax and energize you.

Being overwhelmed is like having a dead battery in your car. The only thing that battery needs is some jumper cables and a quick recharge. Then you can drive your car again, and get back on the road. That's what a theta boost does for you. It restores your energy.

How Does A Boost Of Theta Brainwaves Energize You?

When your body relaxes, your blood pressure drops and your heart rate slows down (or stabilizes) to a comfortable pace. As you relax, you also have more oxygen and blood flow going to the brain. You can think clearly, focus, and remember. When you relax, your brain chemicals naturally elevate your attention span and level of alertness. When your attention span and alertness are high, it is also easier to learn, remember, and memorize. That is why stimulating theta brainwaves is also excellent for ADHD.

Delta: By stimulating delta brainwaves, you will induce sleep. Delta brainwave entrainment is useful for insomnia, as it helps you to relax and fall asleep. Another benefit of increasing your delta brainwaves is that they trigger feelings of empathy, intuition, and awareness. Have you ever thought about someone "out of the blue" and then the phone rang and it was them? Or maybe you had a gut instinct, and this helped you to make a wise decision. This is your delta brainwaves at work. Delta brainwaves can provide you with the ability to read other peoples emotions and understand their feelings at a subconscious level .

Delta brainwaves can help you to read a person's body language, and understand their unspoken cues. You have probably experienced this type of intuition with someone that you care about. You intuitively sense what they are thinking, before they say a word. On a subconscious level, you hear a voice inside your head telling you these things, or maybe you see a mental picture, or have a hunch. All of these things are your delta brainwaves at work.

In healthy amounts, delta brainwaves help you to have an advanced state of empathy, understanding, and compassion for others. If you are intuitive, and sometimes can sense what other people are thinking or feeling, you probably have more delta brainwaves than the average person. On the other hand, if you find that it is difficult to empathize, then you may have less overall delta brainwave activity.

As you use the ALERT on a regular basis, you definitely experience a boost in your intuition and your ability to recognize gut-level feelings. The more than you become consciously aware of the delta brainwave state, the more you will be aware of intuitive feelings, mental pictures, and nonverbal cues.

Slower Brain Waves Trigger The Release Of Neurotransmitters

It is a curious phenomenon. Slower brainwave frequencies (such as delta, theta and alpha) help to produce neurotransmitters in the brain. Slower brainwaves boost the production of serotonin, dopamine, and other neurotransmitters in the brain.

The principles of neuroscience tell us that brain cells are electrochemically triggered to produce certain neurotransmitters, neuropeptides, and hormones at certain brainwave frequencies (Kandel, Schwartz & Jessell, 2000). Your brain cells are activated to produce certain neurochemicals when they are interacting with certain brainwave frequencies. All of this electro-chemical interaction takes place in the brain. When you stimulate your brainwaves, you stimulate the production of healthy neurochemicals, which restore the mind and body to equilibrium.

When you relax with the ALERT, you are encouraging your brainwaves to slow down, rest, and rejuvenate. You are also sending a direct message to your brain that it's time to release the neurochemicals that you need to restore balance to your mind and body.

Actually, the same thing happens when you get a good night's sleep. While you're sleeping, your brain produces many beneficial healing hormones and neurotransmitters. If you wake up feeling well-rested, your energy supply was replenished by the delta and theta brain waves. Sleeping replenished the energy that you need to take charge of your day.

Of course, we don't always feel like this. Sometimes, we awaken feeling groggy, lethargic, and stuck in sleep mode. This could be caused by stress. When you're stressed out, stress hormones (oxytocin, insulin and adrenaline) are being released in your body. If you don't get rid of the stress (with physical exercise or deep relaxation) then the stress chemicals will continually pump into your body, without shutting off. Yes, stress chemicals are produced even when you're asleep. These stress hormones ravage the body day and night, 24/7, forcing your adrenal glands to work overtime. It's a dangerous position to be in.

If you're feeling lethargic when you wake up, this may also be related to theta or delta brainwaves. You might be parked in these brainwaves and stuck there. Ideally, you also want to "get in and out of park" and make a smooth transition between activities. Whenever you have a smooth transition between brainwave states, it is easier for you to get focused, on track, and to gain momentum with the task at hand.

There are four different brainwave frequencies, and each one has something useful to offer. Your brainwaves can enhance your ability to learn, speak, think, and respond. Your brainwaves can make the difference between getting things done and giving up. That is why your brainwaves are an important tool to success.

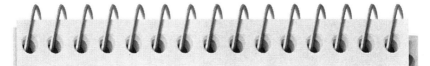

Dear Reader,

Let's take a closer look at what happens when you use the ALERT. Just for fun, let's take a look at the process using popular song lyrics. Here is how the ALERT trains your brain from start to finish:

(1) "Wake me up, before you go go!" Remember when the British pop duo "Wham!" sang this song back in 1984? Picture your sleepy ADHD brain waking up from a deep sleep. A beautiful rhythm has captured your attention. It's the Rhythm of Peak Performance.

(2) "Let's dance!" David Bowie says, "Put on your red shoes and dance the blues" in his 1983 hit. Likewise, your brain is stepping on to the dance floor. Your brain is dancing to the sights and sounds of the ALERT. Your brainwaves are getting into rhythm with the beat.

(3) "We interrupt this program!" A British electronic band named Coburn released this glitchy dance tune in 2005. The song is reminiscent of the sights and sounds of the ALERT interrupting your regularly scheduled programming of ADHD. Unfortunately, ADHD keeps you parked in a dysfunctional rhythm.

(Continued)

The ALERT steps in and interrupts your ADHD. Your brain realizes, "Whoa, we're doing things a little differently now... but I'm ok with that!"

(4) "That's the way, uh huh, I like it!" Your brain is caught up in the dance, just like KC & The Sunshine Band's disco hit from the 1970's. The rhythm gently nudges your brainwaves in the direction of healthier balance. If your brainwaves are too slow, the rhythm speeds up your brainwaves. If your brainwaves are too fast, the rhythm slows down your brainwaves. Gradually, the tempo of your brainwaves is balanced, fine-tuned, and stabilized.

(5) "Talk to me..." Annie Lennox and the Eurythmics sang "Here Comes the Rain Again" in the '80s. The song is about intimate conversation. In the same way, the sights and sounds of the ALERT stimulate your brain cells to talk to each other. As a result, your brain changes electro-chemically. Your brain cells are wiring and firing at a stable pace. Your dendrites are becoming thicker and denser. This enables you to think faster and smarter. Your brain produces a stable supply of neurotransmitters, which helps you to focus and pay attention. As more connections (or synapses) are created in the brain, you develop a greater capacity for transmitting messages and processing information.

(Continued)

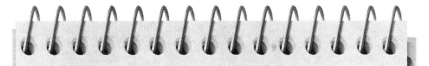

(6) "Walk this way..." Remember Aerosmith's rock song from the 70s? Picture the sights and sounds of the ALERT coaxing your brain: "Don't walk the road of ADHD! Instead, walk this way. Take the path of peak performance." Your brain is rhythmically coaxed in the right direction. As you relax with the sights and sounds of the ALERT, your brain creates new neural pathways.

Over time, these pathways become smoother and more defined. Like an often-traveled path in the woods, the Rhythm of Peak Performance becomes automatic and comfortable.

(7) "Beat it!" Wouldn't it be cool if Michael Jackson's 80's hit was about your brain telling ADHD to beat it because it's not welcome anymore? With the ALERT, your ADHD is like a coward who has lost the fight. Plus, your old ADHD brain map is no longer used. Your new neural pathways become stronger, and your old ADHD ways (distraction, disorganization, restless energy, etc.) fade away. Now, you can access your new and improved state of mind, which is peak performance. As a result, your ability to concentrate, focus, listen, read and remember improves— and your life is transformed.

All the best,
Nicky

CHAPTER 11

Getting Into The Rhythm of Peak Performance

"I twisted my knee while teaching a fitness class. I wanted to keep on exercising, but couldn't do much of anything. A friend suggested that I step up and down on a Coke crate. I worked up a bunch of moves and started teaching this workout at Gold's Gym. A lady in my Step class who worked at Reebok corporate helped me to present my idea to Reebok. My knees were knocking together under the table, when they said they were going to do it. Yes, Reebok picked up my Step routine in 1989, and the rest is history. They thought it might be the next big fitness craze."
— Gin Miller (2009), founder of Step Aerobics, in an interview with Group Fitness Radio.

Let's take a break from the topic of brain training and have some fun. What do you like to do for fun? I like to go to exercise classes at the gym.

One of my favorite classes is Body Step. It's the craziest thing. Everyone gets a rectangular plastic box. The music starts and we're stepping on the box. We step to the left, right, up, and down. The routine speeds up, and so does the footwork. We're doing an "L" step, trotting over the top of the box, and kicking to the left and right. We leap over the box, and do the same routine facing the back of the room. We add a jumping jack, a quick punch, and another kick. Now we're doing the moon walk over the top, straddling the box, jumping off, and then jogging back around.

Whew, it's a fast workout! If I don't pay careful attention, I might trip, fall down, or mess up. I really need to stay on top of this game. It's important to stay "in synch" with the music and the rest of the class. That is what step class is all about.

Of course, I wasn't always up to speed. My first step class was a disaster! I was huffing and puffing to keep up. Just when I mastered the moves on the right, the routine switched to the left. I felt totally out of place, awkward, and clumsy.

It's funny, now that I think about it! Being a newcomer at Step class was a lot like ADHD. There was a mismatch between what I was doing and how my brain works. Everyone else stepped in rhythm with the music. I was out-of-synch and falling all over myself.

Back then, I wondered, "How could I possibly master this routine?" I took a deep breath, and looked around the room. Did other steppers have a special skill or talent that I lacked? Surely, they weren't that much different from me. We all have arms, legs and feet... but we moved at a different pace. Maybe it was just a matter of practice. The other steppers came to class regularly and practiced the routine. Surely, I could do the same!

At the next class, I set my box close to the front, and paid careful attention. I tried to copy (or mirror) the teacher's moves. My eyes were glued to the teacher, and I did exactly what he was doing. I counted the repetitions, and followed the steps in the routine. For instance, the routine involved four steps on the left, and then repeating the same pattern on the right. I counted silently to myself, as I did the steps. This helped me to break down the routine into smaller chunks. To my amazement, I started to catch on and keep the pace. The more I practiced the routine, the easier it became. After a while, the movements seemed to come automatically, without me thinking about it.

As I continued to practice, the step routine became easier and easier. What a difference from my early days of being uncoordinated and clumsy. I wasn't an outsider anymore. Finally, I was up to speed and in-synch with the class. What made the difference? Practice. Doing the same steps over and over again. Plus, paying careful attention to the teacher. He did the routine correctly, and all I needed to do was copy him. It's like they say: Practice makes perfect, and repetition builds mastery.

Step class and the human brain

At step class, there is music playing the background. The music helps the class to follow the rhythm and keep up the tempo or pace. In the same way, there is a rhythm to peak performance. There is a rhythm to focusing, concentrating, and remembering. If you have ADHD, you aren't in-synch with this rhythm. ADHD causes you to be distracted, disorganized, and perform below your abilities.

Plus, with ADHD, certain areas of your brain are weak, lethargic, or unbalanced. Your brainwaves might be too slow (sluggish) or too fast (hyperactive). Plus, you may not have enough juice (neurotransmitters) for your brain to work properly. You may also have low arousal and need a jump start.

The good news is that you can train your brain and transform your life. Whenever you use the ALERT, you practice the Rhythm of Peak Performance. Actually, the scientific name for it is the Sensory Motor Rhythm. For now, let's call it the Rhythm of Peak Performance—because that phrase describes the intended outcome. It is a rhythm that stimulates and arouses the sleepy ADHD brain. It is a rhythm that stabilizes the tempo of your brainwaves and boosts your brain's production of neurotransmitters. It sounds complicated, but it's really a simple process. Let's take a closer look at what happens when you use the ALERT.

How The ALERT Trains Your Brain, From Start To Finish

1. **Your brain is stimulated with the audio-visual rhythm.** This is the first thing that happens when you use the ALERT. Your brain is being stimulated through your eyes and ears. With your eyeglasses, you will see mild flashing lights. With your headphones, you will hear mild heartbeat sounds. In this way, your brain is presented with an audio-visual rhythm that catches your attention. Of course, you're lying flat on your back, with your eyes closed. You may fall asleep or zone out. That doesn't matter. What matters is that your brain is being stimulated with this audio-visual rhythm.

2. **Your brain is challenged.** The ALERT's audio-visual rhythm gently challenges your brain to let go of existing neural patterns, or old ADHD habits. There is a gentle, unspoken challenge to "come dance with me!" In a way, what is about to happen is a lot like a dance. The ALERT's rhythm challenges you to try something different. For the longest time, you've been stuck in a rut with ADHD. You can't seem to break out of your old

habits and patterns. Your brain always goes back to the same old way of doing things. You have been locked into old ADHD habits, and doing the same thing for years. The ALERT's audio-visual rhythm wakes up the sluggish ADHD brain, and challenges you to try a new and exciting rhythm.

3. **Your brain gets in rhythm with the beat.** The audio-visual rhythm of the ALERT is different from anything that you've ever experienced before. This new rhythm is fun, and your brain likes it. Your brain starts to dance with the rhythm. Yes, you're still lying on your back, with your eyes closed, but your brain is stepping out on the dance floor.

You might be wondering, "How is this possible? Is my brain really dancing?" Yes, that's exactly what's happening. Your brain is dancing to the rhythm that it is hearing and seeing. Your brain is mirroring, mimicking, or getting in-synch with that rhythm. This phenomenon is known as entrainment.

It's the same thing that happens when you hear your favorite song on the radio. You might move your head, snap your fingers, or tap your feet. You're getting into rhythm with the music. In the same way, your brain gets in rhythm with the sights and sounds of the ALERT. Even if you're lying flat and motionless on your back, your brain is dancing along with the rhythm.

4. **Your brain copies the rhythm.** Have you ever attended a sporting event where the crowd does a big wave? Perhaps you've done this at a football game, or some other event. Usually, the wave starts out slow, with the one section of the crowd raising their arms up, and then down. The next section of the crowd does the same thing, and the wave goes all around the stadium. The crowd usually repeats the wave a second time, but faster. The wave goes faster and faster. Your brain is like that.

When you use the ALERT, your brain is copying the rhythm it hears and sees. When the rhythm goes faster, your brainwaves go faster. When the rhythm slows down, your brainwaves slow down. Your brainwaves are following the rhythm perfectly. Your brain translates the ALERT's audio-visual rhythm into electrical impulses or brainwaves. Your brain gets into rhythm with the beat. Your brain's electrical impulses travel from one brain cell to another, like a crowd doing the wave at a football game.

5. Your brain's self-regulating system is interrupted. Your brain has a wonderful self-regulating system. It is constantly striving for balance and equilibrium. Unfortunately, ADHD has messed things up. Your brainwaves are parked in a dysfunctional rhythm. The problem has gotten so bad that your brain considers the ADHD rhythm to be normal. However, something magical happens when you're exposed to the sights and sounds of the ALERT. Your brain's firing patterns are gently nudged in the direction of a healthier balance. This nudging interrupts the brain's self-regulating system. Your brain says, "Whoa, we're doing things a little differently now... and I'm ok with that!" Occasionally, your brain may push back, and resist the rapid change. That is why consistent, daily training with the ALERT is so important, especially with the first 60 days.

6. The tempo of your brainwaves is stabilized. If your brainwaves are too slow, the rhythm speeds up your brainwaves. If your brainwaves are too fast, the rhythm slows down your brainwaves. Gradually, the tempo of your brainwaves is balanced, fine-tuned, and stabilized. This happens automatically as you get in-synch with the sights and sounds of the ALERT. The rhythm balances your brainwaves, so that the tempo is within a normal range.

7. Your brain teaches itself to normalize. As your brain gets in-synch with the Rhythm of Peak Performance, it gradually becomes comfortable. It's as if your brain realizes, "I like this! Yes, this is the rhythm that I'm dancing to now." Your brain teaches itself to hold and maintain the new Rhythm of Peak Performance. This is a big change for the brain's self-regulating system. The Rhythm of Peak Performance becomes the new auto-pilot.

8. Your brain begins to change electro-chemically. Your brain cells are firing and wiring. Your dendrites, or "magic trees of the mind," become thicker and denser. This enables you to think faster and smarter. Your brain starts to produce a stable supply of neurotransmitters, which helps you to focus and pay attention. The more you use the ALERT, the more connections (or synapses) are created in the brain. This gives you a greater capacity for transmitting messages and processing information, which translates to higher intelligence and better mental functioning.

9. **Your brain is conditioned.** Every time you use the ALERT, you are practicing the Rhythm of Peak Performance. You are reinforcing and solidifying the neural connections in your brain. Eventually, this process becomes completely automatic, and you're able to hold this rhythm for longer periods of time, until the rhythm becomes permanent.

10. **Your brain creates a new brain map.** With repeated practice, your neural pathways become stronger and more solidified. You are literally changing the structure and patterns in your brain. Sometimes, this process is called "rewiring the brain." You are creating a new brain map for learning.

With the ALERT, your ADHD is like a coward who has lost the fight. Your old ADHD brain map is no longer used. Your new neural pathways become stronger, and your old ADHD ways (distraction, disorganization, restless energy, etc.) fade away. Now you can access your new and improved state of mind, which is peak performance. As a result, your ability to concentrate, focus, listen, read and remember improves— and your life is transformed.

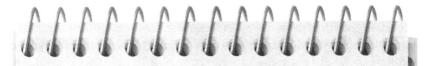

Dear Reader,

The brain training process can be summed up in one word: Entrainment. Perhaps you already understand what this means. To entrain means to follow a rhythm and move at the same pace. The ALERT uses entrainment to train your brain for peak performance.

With the ALERT, entrainment is what happens when your brain dances (or gets in-synch) with the rhythm it is seeing and hearing. It is a phenomenon that happens automatically, without conscious effort.

The power of entrainment is what helps you to train your brain and transform your life. What a difference from Ritalin, which is temporary, and fails to make any permanent changes in the brain. The ALERT's brainwave entrainment literally changes the structure and patterns in your brain. This process is called re-writing the brain. These changes are permanent, and they're yours to keep.

"Your gains will be sustained," says Dr. Paul Swingle (2008), in his book Biofeedback for the Brain: How Neurotherapy Effectively Treats Depression, ADHD, Autism, And More.

(Continued)

Dr. Swingle makes this statement about neuro-feedback (another form of brain training) but it's also true about the ALERT. When you complete the 60-day ALERT program, you should be able to keep the gains you've made.

Dr. Swingle says the only thing that will cause you to regress is trauma. Of course, trauma could be anything: Losing your job, ending a relationship, being in a car accident, a bitter argument, or a crisis.

If your brainwaves become dysfunctional for any reason, they may not return to a normal healthy balance after the event has passed.

Of course, that's when the ALERT can help you. If you're having a bad ADHD day, or struggling with stress, just take time out for an ALERT session. It only takes 22 minutes to do a session, and it's an excellent way to relax, de-stress, and gently stimulate your brain.

With the ALERT, you have an easy-to-use tool that enables you to conquer your ADHD. And when you train your brain, you also transform your life.

All the best,
Nicky

CHAPTER 12

Unleashing The Power Of Brainwave Entrainment

"You know what music is? God's little reminder that there's something else besides us in this universe. It's a harmonic connection between all living beings, every where, even the stars. The music is all around you, all you have to do is listen." —From the movie, "August Rush" (2007).

"Entrainment is not an everyday word, but it's a term used in various fields of science. It can describe the phenomenon of one organism rhythmically and internally adjusting itself to another. It's when life pulses coordinate. Fireflies lighting up in synchronization has been described as entrainment. Jazz musicians locking in together is, in a way, entrainment." —Ben Ratliff (2009), in his music review for the *New York Times*.

In the last chapter, we talked about the sights and sounds of the ALERT, and how this rhythm trains your brain for peak performance. Part of the magic that makes this work is entrainment. It's a scientific term, but it doesn't have to be complicated. To entrain means to follow a rhythm and move at the same pace. It's like the step class mentioned in the last chapter. A group of people stepping on boxes in rhythm with music is an example of entrainment.

With the ALERT, entrainment is what happens when your brain dances (or gets in-synch) with the rhythm it is seeing and hearing. It is a phenomenon that happens automatically, without conscious effort. Another word for entrainment is "synchrony." Synch means "together" and chrony means "in time." Literally, synchrony means together in time, or moving at the same pace.

Entrainment also refers to a steady pace, tempo, or beat. More specifically, an entrained rhythm helps you to achieve a specific outcome. In step class, the music is an entrained rhythm that helps you to learn the routine. The sights and sounds of the ALERT are entrained rhythms that help you to conquer ADHD.

The "light and sound" industry is all about brainwave entrainment (BWE). Sometimes, it is called Audio-Visual Brainwave Entrainment (AVE) or Audio-Visual Stimulation (AVS).

The concept of entrainment is important because it helps us understand the rhythmic quality of the human brain. Entrainment is what enables us to stimulate and arouse the brain, the same way that Ritalin does, without swallowing pills. The power of entrainment is what helps you to train your brain and transform your life.

Entrainment: Here, There And Everywhere

Entrainment is a commonly accepted principle that appears in biology, chemistry, medicine, astronomy, and psychology. It also occurs with the human brain. Here are some examples.

Biology. Frogs make a repetitive, pulse-like, croaking sound. It is a rhythm that is driven by the neural connections in the frog's brain. A bunch of frogs will croak in unison, as if making music. This is an example of mutual entrainment. The frogs lock into this mutual rhythm, and croak at the same pitch and tempo. The same thing happens with crickets, birds, and other animals. Many animals make similar sounds as a group, creating harmony, and locking into a mutual rhythm.

Have you ever been to an aquarium, and watched a school of fish swim in unison? Every tail and fin swishes in rhythm with the rest of the group. The rhythm has a musical quality to it. These fish are entrained to swim together in perfect harmony. Why do they swim together like that? The main reason is survival. There is strength in numbers. A school of fish has a greater chance of survival in the open sea than a single fish.

When a predator looks for food, the school of fish gives the appearance of being a big fish and the predator may think twice about going after them for dinner. Meanwhile, a single fish is not a threat, and may be gobbled up without a second thought.

Have you ever looked up to the sky, and watched a flock of birds fly in a "V" formation? The rhythm and synchronized flying is an example of entrainment. Flying this way creates a "slip stream" effect which lowers air resistance and makes it easier for the flock of birds to fly long distances. As a flock, they don't have to expend as much energy as if they were flying solo.

Chemistry. Honeybees work together to make honey. Each bee works in synchronicity with the rest of their colony. Honeybees produce enzymes that turn the nectar gathered from flowers into sucrose, glucose, and fructose. The bees must work together in a rhythmic harmony to order to achieve the unique chemical composition of honey.

Medicine. Perhaps you've visited someone in the hospital who was using a nebulizer. It is a mouthpiece that enables them to inhale oxygen or liquid medication in mist form. The nebulizer features an "entrainment dial"—a knob that provides a steady, simultaneous flow of mist. The entrainment enables the nebulizer to deliver the mist at a stable and continuous pace.

Entrainment In The Human Body

In the human body, all vital functions are rhythmic. There are biological rhythms involved in body temperature, blood pressure, heart rate, mental alertness, hormone secretion, neurotransmitter production, physical strength, aerobic capacity/oxygen intake, digestion, and countless other functions of the human body. There is even a rhythm to the hair that grows on your head. These are all examples of entrained rhythms in the body. In other words, there is a tempo to all of these body functions that helps to create a specific outcome.

Sometimes, the rhythms of the human body are described as "circadian rhythms." Your body's internal clock completes a rhythmic cycle every 24 hours in synchrony with the eternal clock of the earth's rotation—the day and night cycle. The rhythms of the human body enable it to achieve balance, or homeostasis.

Interestingly, the human body is always working on balancing these rhythms. Consider what happens when you exercise. You work up a sweat, and your heart beats faster. As the sweat evaporates from your skin, you cool down and your body temperature returns to normal. Your body also attempts to stabilize your heart rate and returns it to a normal resting rate. This is the power of homeostasis at work.

More Examples Of Homeostasis

Your body also stabilizes your blood pressure. If your blood pressure is too high or low, your body automatically attempts to restore it to normal levels. When you have a fever, your body attempts to get sickness out of your system, and return to a state of homeostasis. If you're hungry, you will crave food to eat. Why? So that you will have enough energy to get through the day. Your body is working towards equilibrium so that you can be healthy. It's interesting that your internal rhythms are helping you to achieve this balance. Almost all of your bodily functions are rhythmic, entrained, and strive to maintain balance. The more stable and balanced your body rhythms are, the better you will feel.

You might be thinking, "All of this is fine, but my mind and body aren't always perfect." That's true. You wouldn't have ADHD, if your mind and body were in a state of perfect equilibrium.

We've already talked about why ADHD occurs: Weak electro-chemical communication in the brain, dopamine deficiency, slow brainwaves, and "low arousal" because you're not getting enough stimulation. All of these things reflect a lack of equilibrium in the brain. Unfortunately, there was a point where ADHD took over, and bad habits like distraction and disorganization became the norm. With ADHD, your brain no longer re-sets, or returns to the homeostasis of concentrating, focusing and remembering.

Instead of homeostatis, your ADHD brain creates allostasis— a term used by neuroscientist Bruce McEwen (2002) in his book, *The End of Stress As We Know It.*

McEwen (2002) uses the term allostasis to describe a stress response in which the mind and body turns against itself. When this happens, your production of new brain cells is cut in half, and maximum energy is delivered to those parts of the mind and body that are critical for self-protection. This is a reasonable explanation as to why your brain works to maintain ADHD. Your mind and body have turned against themselves.

Your brain will always take the fastest, shortest route. Usually, that means doing things the same way you've done them before. It is like water trickling down a rock. The water is mostly likely going to follow the grooves that are already in the rock (rather than making new ones).

"We Interrupt This Regularly Scheduled Program...."

Have you ever watched TV, and your show was interrupted? The announcer says, "We interrupt our regularly scheduled program to bring you this special announcement." Usually, it's weather information or updates on political elections.

An interruption is the last thing you want when you're watching your favorite TV show. But interruptions are a good thing for ADHD. An interruption is exactly what your brain needs in order to make a change, and move away from the way things were done before. Your brain cells need to go a different route, and a new pathway is created in the brain. This new path must be taken repeatedly, so that it becomes paved and established. That's when the old road is no longer used. New synapses are formed between brain cells, and the old path is pruned away (Mahoney & Restak, 1988; Hawley, 2000; Sprenger 1999; Kandel 2007).

With ADHD, your brainwaves are stuck (or parked) in a dysfunctional rhythm. Your brainwaves may be sluggish (too slow) or hyperactive (too fast), or somewhere in between. The ALERT's brainwave entrainment gently challenges your brain to let go of the dysfunctional rhythm. It corrects the imbalance, so that the speed of your brainwaves is within a normal range. The Rhythm of Peak Performance interrupts the old ADHD pattern with a new rhythm that creates new neural pathways in the brain. Eventually, your old brain map of ADHD is replaced with a new brain map.

You Can Reset Your Brain's Rhythms

Scientists have discovered that our circadian rhythms can be reset (Kandel, Schwartz & Jessell, 2000). Yes, it's scientific, but it is also common sense. For example, consider jet lag. If you get on a plane and cross time zones, you will probably feel woozy and fatigued. After all, your old rhythm is different than the one you're currently experiencing. There is a different time zone, which forces you to change the time you wake up and go to sleep. Often, this time change makes you lethargic and disoriented. In a few days, however, your body quickly readjusts and the jet lag goes away. Previously, your biological clock had you going to sleep and waking up at a different time. Now, your brain must reset your body's rhythms. You're in a different time zone, and you must get up and go to sleep at a different time. There is an adjustment in the day and night, sleep and waking time clock, and you must adjust to the current time zones.

Another example of resetting brain rhythms is the readjustment made by people who work at night. This disrupts their regular sleep schedule. People who work at night tend to sleep during the day. Of course, sleeping during the day disrupts their regular schedule and circadian rhythms. But, it is possible to reset these rhythms. It might take a little while, but night workers will eventually get accustomed to working at night and sleeping during the day. By doing so, they have reset their brain's rhythms.

In the same way, you can reset the rhythms of ADHD. With ADHD, you may be locked into a pattern of being distracted and disorganized. ADHD is a glitch that undermines your ability to concentrate, focus and remember. It is as if you're "rhythmically challenged."

Do you remember the movie "Mr. Holland's Opus?" Richard Dreyfuss played a band director who taught high school students to play instruments and march at the same time. A couple of students were rhythmically challenged. They were clumsy and uncoordinated, but practice enabled them to get up to speed. What changed their rhythm? Practice and repetition. The students practiced until they were able to march and play their instruments at the same time.

In the same way, ADHD causes us to be rhythmically challenged. We're out of synch with the Rhythm of Peak Performance. We haven't mastered that rhythm, and this makes it difficult for us to concentrate, focus, and get organized.

The key to mastery is practicing the rhythm over and over again. Practice makes perfect, and repetition builds mastery. When you use the ALERT, you are exposed to the Rhythm of Peak Performance (or Sensory Motor Rhythm). This rhythm gently nudges your brainwaves in a healthy direction. If your brainwaves are too slow, then the rhythm speeds up your brainwaves, If your brainwaves are too fast, then the rhythm slows down your brainwaves. Gradually, the tempo of your brainwaves becomes stabilized. This happens automatically as you get in-synch with the sights and sounds of the ALERT. The rhythm balances your brainwaves, so the tempo is within a normal range.

Daily practice will help you achieve rhythmic integration and balance to your brain. The light and sound technology acts an entraining signal. Practicing the Rhythm of Peak Performance has a dramatic effect on your ability to concentrate, focus, and stay on track.

The brainwave entrainment of the ALERT allows you to accomplish a lot. Actually, there is more to it than simply following a rhythm and moving at the same pace. Consider these ten things that entrainment does for your brain.

The ALERT's Brainwave Entrainment Teaches Your Brain To:

1. **Restore and repair itself.** The brainwave entrainment of the ALERT stimulates the neural circuits in the brain. This is best done with a combination of light and sound stimulation directed toward smaller, deficient brain circuits. Ultimately, the stimulation of these weaker areas makes your brain stronger, more flexible, and efficient. The brainwave entrainment also helps to boost neurotransmitter levels (such as dopamine) so that you can think clearly, concentrate, and focus.

2. **Tame and normalize any irregular brain rhythms.** With ADHD, your brain is like a wild animal: Easily distracted, disorganized, and impulsive. Your brainwaves may be out-of-control, irregular, and unstable. Unfortunately, your brain is parked in a dysfunctional ADHD rhythm. The ALERT gently challenges your brain to let go of these existing neural patterns and try something new. It uses brainwave entrainment to stabilize brainwaves that are sluggish or hyperactive. Brainwave entrainment with the ALERT helps to correct this imbalance, so that the speed of your brainwaves is within a normal range.

3. **Move towards harmony and homeostasis.** Harmony is always better than disharmony. The brainwave entrainment of the ALERT facilitates harmony (rhythmic integration) and homeostasis (balance). The more integrated your rhythms, the better you feel.

4. **Quicken your mental processing and response time.** It is important for your brain cells to go in and out of rest quickly. As you open and close your eyes, your brain must make a quick transition from rest to being ready for activity.

People with ADHD tend to be adrenaline junkies. There is a rush of adrenaline that comes from a thrill-seeking activity. The feel-good adrenaline rush gives you the juice that you need to focus and get ready for action. Thrill seeking also quickens your response time—so that you respond faster to the task in front of you. The ALERT uses brainwave entrainment to boost arousal, so that you can naturally achieve a natural state of readiness.

5. **Gain momentum.** The brainwave entrainment of the ALERT teaches you a rhythm that helps you to gain momentum. With ADHD, you're easily distracted, and tend to stop and start over many times. Or you may put things off, or don't finish what you start. As a result, it takes longer to get things done. The brainwave entrainment of the ALERT helps you to get a rhythm going, so that you can stay focused until you're finished. Finally, you can get your life going in the right direction and build momentum. Brainwave entrainment helps you to get busy creating the life you want.

6. **Quiet your inner dialogue.** The brainwave entrainment of the ALERT has a calming effect that soothes your ADHD. As you entrain to the sights and sounds of the ALERT, you will experience a relaxed state of mind. If you have ADHD, you have a tendency to be stressed out, anxious, and distracted. Plus, your mind chatters. This makes it difficult for you to think clearly, get organized and finish your work. But something magical happens with the ALERT. As your brain entrains to the rhythm, your mind chatter begins to slow down and ease up. As a result, you become calm and tranquil. You can let go of tension and anxiety. As a result, you're able to think more clearly and creatively. The calm state of mind also enhances your awareness, intuition, and problem solving ability.

7. **Improve your blood circulation and oxygen intake.** The brain-wave entrainment of the ALERT helps to increase the amount of oxygen going to your brain. Oxygen is the fuel for all the activities in the brain that lead to high thinking. A stable supply of oxygen helps you to think clearly and respond quickly.

The ALERT also increases blood flow to the brain. This is important because your blood cells carry oxygen to your brain and other organs. The brain accounts for more than 25 percent of the body's blood flow (Kandel, Schwartz & Jessell, 2000). Without adequate blood flow, your brain is deprived of oxygen and thus is unable to operate at peak efficiency (Sears, 2008). Your brain cells are designed to receive stimulation, and the boost that they receive from the ALERT (improved blood circulation and oxygen intake) results in healthy growth and change.

8. **Create automatic behaviors of improved concentration, focus, and memory.** The ALERT creates brainwave entrainment that encourages the brain to grow new neural connections and release neurotransmitters. As your brain cells become stronger and more efficient at talking to each other, you will experience a significant improvement in your ability to concentrate, focus and remember. Best of all, these behaviors become automatic. You won't have to think about it or get motivated. It is like riding a bike or driving a car. Once you learn it, you can do it easily and effortlessly, without thinking too much about it.

9. **Practice and master the Rhythm of Peak Performance.** The quickest way to learn something is practice. You can practice something repeatedly, until you get it right. When you use the ALERT, you will hear and see the Rhythm of Peak Performance. In response, your brain practices the rhythm that it is hearing and seeing. Your brain entrains with this rhythm. As a result, you create new neural pathways and brain maps. Your old ADHD behaviors eventually fade away. Your ADHD will be replaced with the Rhythm of Peak Performance. Finally, you can break the habit of ADHD once and for all!

10. **Make permanent, lasting changes in the brain... for the better!** The ALERT is different from Ritalin, which only lasts four to eight hours, and fails to make any permanent changes in the brain. The ALERT's brainwave entrainment literally changes the structure and

patterns in your brain. This process is called re-writing the brain. These changes are permanent, and they're yours to keep.

"Your gains will be sustained," says Dr. Paul Swingle (2008), in his book *Biofeedback for the Brain: How Neurotherapy Effectively Treats Depression, ADHD, Autism, and More.*

Dr. Swingle made this statement about neurofeedback (another form of brain training) but it is also true about the ALERT. When you complete the 60-day ALERT program, you should be able to keep the gains you've made. Dr. Swingle says the only thing that will cause you to regress is trauma. Of course, trauma could be anything: Losing your job, ending a relationship, being in a car accident, a bitter argument, or a crisis. If your brainwaves become dysfunctional for any reason, they may not return to a normal healthy balance after the event has passed.

If you experience trauma, the ALERT is always there to help you. If you're having a bad ADHD day, or struggling with stress, just take time out for an ALERT session. It only takes 22 minutes to do a session, and it's an excellent way to relax, de-stress and gently stimulate your brain. With the ALERT, you have an easy-to-use tool that enables you to conquer your ADHD.

Be Prepared

Let me close this chapter with a personal story. My family and I went to Carowinds, a local amusement park. It was a warm sunny day, but suddenly the skies grew dark and it started to rain. My husband Jim reached into his book bag and pulled out four plastic ponchos, packed down to the size of credit cards. Our 8-year-old son, Perry, giggled.

"Dad, this reminds me of the Boy Scout motto," said Perry.

"Yep," said Jim. "Always be prepared!"

The same thing is true about ADHD. Bad things can happen when we least expect it, but we can be prepared for the storms of life. How do you respond when things go wrong? You probably have some tools for coping—such as prayer, your faith, and the support of family and friends. Perhaps you use positive psychology, such as affirmations, positive thinking, having a confident expectation, goal setting, and taking action. You may also exercise, eat healthy foods, and occasionally get a massage. The ALERT is a wonderful addition to those tools.

You can use the ALERT to let go of stress and anxiety. You can use the ALERT when you feel restless, and crave a little extra burst of energy. You can also use the ALERT to stimulate and arouse your brain. You can use the ALERT to boost your ability to focus and get things done.

Isn't that better than running to the medicine cabinet when you have a headache or feel stressed out? The ALERT is a natural, drug-free way to cope with the stress and strains of life. It will help you to be prepared for whatever comes your way. And when you train your brain, you also transform your life.

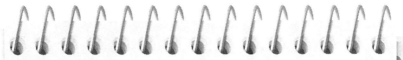

Dear Reader,

While researching this book, I found a treasure buried deep in the scientific literature. It was practically hidden from public view. I'd never heard of it before, and you probably haven't either. It's more valuable than gold or silver, especially for folks with ADHD. What is it? The Sensory Motor Rhythm (or SMR).

The SMR is the key to conquering ADHD without drugs. It's a natural way to train your brain for peak performance.

The SMR was discovered in the late 1960s, by a neuroscientist named Dr. Barry Sterman. He discovered this brainwave frequency which enabled stray cats to concentrate and tune out distractions. When this brainwave frequency is reached, the cat's brain communicated with their body's motor systems to settle down, tune out distractions, and tap into their body's natural energy—which is a state of calm. Dr. Sterman called it the Sensory Motor Rhythm.

In his college laboratory, Dr. Sterman used the SMR to train the cats to remain calm, exercise self-control, withhold their response, and show motor stillness. The cats even ignored the distraction of food and water with the SMR.

(Continued)

In the 1970s, Dr. Sterman took his research a step further. He was approached by a woman who worked in his lab. Her name was Margaret Fairbanks.

Ms. Fairbanks watched Dr. Sterman do amazing things with the stray cats. She wondered if the doctor would test the SMR on her. She suffered from epilepsy, and desperately wanted to be cured. At the time, Ms. Fairbanks couldn't drive a car. Evidently, epileptics were not allowed to obtain a driver's license. As you can imagine, It was a real hassle not being able to drive. Ms. Fairbanks dreamed of getting her driver's license. Could Dr. Sterman make her dreams come true?

Dr. Sterman agreed to experiment on Ms. Fairbanks. He used the same SMR treatment on Ms. Fairbanks that he used with the stray cats. Ultimately, the SMR training enabled Ms. Fairbanks to change her brainwaves and reduce her tendency to have seizures. She checked with her doctor, and was found to be no longer epileptic! Finally, Ms. Fairbanks was able to get her driver's license (Sterman 1978; Demos, 2005). It was a dream come true!

It didn't take long for other researchers to ask: "If you can change the brainwaves of a person with epilepsy, then why not change the brainwaves of a person with ADHD?"

(Continued)

Dr. Sterman looked for ways to test the Sensory Motor Rhythm on people with ADHD. He met with Drs. Joel and Judith Lubar, who are psychology professors at the University of Tennessee.

Dr. Sterman worked with the Lubars to apply the concept of the SMR to ADHD. The Lubars used the SMR to teach children to pay attention, focus, concentrate, and be less distracted. They taught children with ADHD to be more resistant to attentional lapses and hyperactive outbursts.

The Lubars were able to reduce ADHD symptoms by stabilizing the children's brainwave patterns with the Sensory Motor Rhythm.

Ultimately, the Sensory Motor Rhythm launched the field of neurofeedback. Today, it is used in brain training clinics across the country to help people train their brains to conquer ADHD. Now you can practice and master this same rhythm in the comfort of your own home, without ever stepping foot inside a clinic. The ALERT enables you to practice and master the SMR until it becomes an automatic response. When you master the Sensory Motor Rhythm, your ADHD will be replaced with the Rhythm of Peak Performance.

All the best,
Nicky

CHAPTER 13

Unleashing The Sensory Motor Rhythm

"I hooked up to a neurofeedback instrument for my first session. After training for a half hour, my mind was tired, my thoughts muddled. But an hour or so after I finished, I experienced what is known as the clear windshield effect. The world looked sharp and crystalline, and I had a quiet, energetic feeling that lasted a couple of hours. It was the first time that I had felt that way in years. And it convinced me to look a little deeper. This new biofeedback was something different, I was told, a new technique that could treat Attention Deficit Disorder... and a long list of other problems. I looked into the research and found that the technique had been spawned by solid laboratory research on epilepsy in the 1970s and 1980s." —Jim Robbins (2008), from his book, *A Symphony In The Brain: The Evolution Of The New Brainwave Biofeedback.*

If you did a Google search for the Rhythm of Peak Performance, you'll probably come up empty handed. However, you'll find plenty about this rhythm under its official scientific name: The Sensory Motor Rhythm (or SMR). It is a treatment that is widely used in neurofeedback and brain training clinics throughout the country. The SMR may be the biggest breakthrough in non-invasive medicine in the past 50 years. With the ALERT, you can practice this rhythm in the comfort of your own home, without spending thousands of dollars on treatment, or even a gallon of gas to drive to a clinic.

The SMR is often written about in research journals, and is well-known in neurofeedback circles. However, the public doesn't know much about it, and you probably won't hear about it from your medical doctor. It is a revolutionary rhythm that has been scientifically proven to reduce ADHD. This chapter deals with the discovery of the SMR, and how it was tested and documented. We'll also take a closer look at how the SMR is used in the ALERT sessions to train your brain and transform your life.

What Is The SMR?

The Sensory Motor Rhythm was discovered almost 50 years ago by Dr. Barry Sterman, a neuroscientist at UCLA medical school. It is a brainwave frequency that is associated with motor stillness and calm focus. It is the ability to concentrate without a sense of urgency. The SMR is a beta brainwave frequency of 12 to 15 Hz. When this electrical brainwave frequency is reached, it sets the brain up to communicate with the body's motor systems to settle down, tune out distractions, and tap into your body's natural energy—which is a state of calm.

The SMR also soothes restless energy. It helps to soothe feelings of "I can't stand this a second longer" or "Get me outta here." If you have ADHD, you're familiar with the frustration that comes with waiting in line, listening to a boring speaker, or driving behind a slowpoke. The SMR can rescue you from restless energy. It calms your jittery nerves, so that you can roll with the punches, rather than getting stressed out. It also gives you a stick-to-it-iveness that enables you to focus, concentrate, get organized, and complete assignments in record time.

Discovery Of The SMR

Dr. Sterman discovered the Sensory Motor Rhythm in his laboratory, while experimenting with stray cats. Sterman used the SMR to train the cats to remain calm, exercise self-control, withhold their response, and show motor stillness at 12 to15 Hz brainwave frequencies. The cats even ignored the distraction of food and water with the SMR.

Sternman used certain sounds to activate this brainwave frequency, and he named it the Sensory Motor Rhythm (Roth, Sterman & Clemente, 1967; Sterman & Wywicka, 1967; Wywicka & Sterman, 1968).

Amazingly, the cats used in Dr. Sterman's experiment were not sweet and cuddly house pets. They were stray, undomesticated, feral cats who were born outside. Feral cats usually live in the wild, without human contact. They are not used to being touched, held or handled. Typically, feral cats keep away from people and run away if you try to approach them. Training feral cats is a long process that involves gentle persuasion and a lot of patience. The name feral literally means "wild beast."

SMR, Epilepsy & Margaret Fairbanks

In the 1970s, Dr. Sterman was approached by a staff worker named Margaret Fairbanks. She asked Dr. Sterman to test the SMR on her. Ms. Fairbanks had watched Dr. Sterman do amazing things with the cats, and she wondered if the SMR could reduce her epilepsy. Evidently, she couldn't obtain a driver's license, and it was a real hassle finding a ride to work. (It was assumed that epileptics are more likely to have car accidents, so they are not permitted to drive).

Dr. Sterman agreed to experiment on Ms. Fairbanks. He used the same SMR treatment that he previously used with stray cats. (Sterman, MacDonald & Stone, 1974). The SMR training enabled Ms. Fairbanks to gradually change her brainwaves and reduce her tendency to have seizures. She was no longer considered epileptic. Ms. Fairbanks eventually earned her driver's license, which she was extremely proud of (Demos, 2005).

Implications Of The SMR

The implications of the Sensory Motor Rhythm were mind boggling. Certain sounds could induce brainwave frequencies that created a calm focus, the ability to tune out distractions, and concentrate without a sense of urgency. This SMR was effective in stray cats, and it also helped Margaret Fairbanks recover from epilepsy.

Dr. Sterman continued to work with epileptics. Sterman used brain training (more specifically, neurofeedback) to train people with seizure disorders to produce different brainwaves, so that they could reduce their seizure activity. He demonstrated that people with low brainwave activity (epileptics) could be trained to produce higher frequency brainwaves. Rather than producing excessive brainwaves in the slow 4 to 7 Hz range, they were trained to produce more SMR brainwaves with the frequency of 14 Hz (Sterman & MacDonald & Stone, 1974; Shouse & Sterman, 1979; Sterman & McDonald, 1978; Lantz & Sterman, 1988; Shouse, & Sterman, 1981; Bowersox & Sterman, 1981).

It didn't take long for other researchers to ask: "If you can change the brainwaves of a person with epilepsy, then why not change the brainwaves of a person with ADHD?" (Hill & Castro, 2002).

Dr. Sterman worked with Drs. Joel & Judith Lubar, who are professors of psychology at the University of Tennessee. It took several months to apply the concept of the SMR to ADHD. The Lubars used the SMR to train children to boost the 4 to 7 Hz theta brainwave range and increase their brainwaves to 14 Hz. When children with ADHD received this treatment, they showed a significant reduction in their ADHD symptoms (Lubar & Shouse, 1976; Lubar & Lubar, 1984; Lubar, 1989).

In the 1970s, the Lubars began using the Sensory Motor Rhythm to teach children to pay attention, focus, concentrate, and be less distracted. They taught children with ADHD to be more resistant to attentional lapses and hyperactive outbursts. The Lubars were able to reduce ADHD symptoms by stabilizing the children's brainwave patterns with the SMR.

SMR Boosts Immunity

The Sensory Motor Rhythm was also found to boost immunity (Sterman 1978 & 1979). The SMR may boost the body's immune system, so that it can avoid infection, disease, or toxins.

Dr. Sterman became interested in immunity when NASA asked him to test a toxic rocket fuel called Hydrazine. In his laboratory, Dr. Sterman investigated whether the rocket fuel could cause seizures in stray cats (Sterman, Goodman & Kovalesky, 1978; Sterman & Kovalesky, 1979).

The cats were exposed to the rocket fuel. Half of the cats experienced seizures, but the other half of the cats (those who had increased SMR brainwaves from the last experiment) had a dramatic reduction in their seizure thresholds. The outcome was surprising and unexpected. The SMR appeared to strengthen the cats' immune system, so that they were able to tolerate the toxic fuel.

SMR Launches The Field Of Brain Training

Ultimately, the discovery of the Sensory Motor Rhythm launched the field of brain training. It has been successfully used to treat thousands of people with ADHD. In fact, SMR training is one of the most common protocols for ADHD.

SMR Improves Academic Performance

Researchers have also found the SMR improves academic performance of people with ADHD, and increases scores on the Wechsler Intelligence Scales and the TOVA (Thompson & Thompson, 1998).

Boy Treated With SMR No Longer Needs Special Ed

Psychologists Michael Tansey and Richard Bruner (1983) published a landmark case study in which the SMR was used to help a fourth grade boy with perceptual impairment and hyperactivity. After practicing and mastering the SMR, the boy no longer needed Ritalin. His pediatrician moved the boy out of his special education class into a normal fourth grade classroom, where he improved his grades. Ten years after the completion of treatment, the boy had finished high school and was in college (Tansey, 1993).

To summarize, SMR is a relaxation training that enables you to reduce ADHD by achieving a relaxed focus, improved concentration, enhanced attention span and creativity. Developing this rhythm also soothes restless energy, quiets impulsivity, and minimizes distractions.

SMR Used For Various Health Concerns

The SMR is also used to successfully treat anxiety and depression (Éismont & Aliyeva, 2008); PMS and migraines (Pfurtscheller, 2008), sleep disorders and chronic pain syndrome (Hoedlmoser & Pecherstorfer, 2008), autism (Stroganova & Nygren, 2007), and cerebral palsy (Finley & Niman, 1976).

ADHD & The Brain's Sensory Motor System

Cheryl Chia, a physiotherapist in Bangkok, contends ADHD is caused by the brain's Sensory Motor System not operating efficiently (Johnson & Trivitayakhun, 2010).

Ms. Chia insists that a person's Sensory Motor System must be in perfect sync in order to concentrate, focus and remember. While sitting at a desk, your brain must direct your neck muscles to hold your head steady. Your brain must control your eye movement across the page and focus your eyesight, so that you can see and make sense of the words. Your brain is actively working, whether you're writing by hand or typing on your computer keyboard. The fingers, wrist and forearm must work in unison while the brain is processing and retaining information. All of these things must be in synch in order for you to be productive.

Your brain must also tune out distractions such as the room temperature, background noise, other people, plus the thoughts and cares of the day (coming from your inner dialogue). Evidently, the ability to tune out distractions is also a function of the brain's Sensory Motor System (Johnson & Trivitayakhun, 2010). That is why the SMR is the perfect antidote for ADHD. The SMR gives you to ability to focus and respond quickly, plus tune out distractions.

SMR Calms Restlessness & Hyperactivity

"The SMR is an calming rhythm which resides only in the motor strip of the brain," explains Dave Siever, the Director of Mind Alive, the company which manufactures the ALERT.

"The SMR functions as a calming rhythm in the motor strip, in the same way that alpha brainwaves calm the rest of brain. ADHD children have low SMR activity because they are hyperactive. SMR is under control of the frontal (reasoning and attending) part of the brain, which inhibits the motor strip when it's operating properly. With ADHD, the frontal part is largely sleeping in theta and doesn't inhibit the motor strip. Therefore, the motor strip (and child) becomes hyperactive and the SMR is reduced," explained Mr. Siever.

"When an ADHD child takes a stimulant drug such as Ritalin, the front part of the brain wakes up and calms the motor strip. In turn, the SMR increases and the child relaxes," said Mr. Siever.

With the ALERT, your brain increases its SMR directly from the audio visual stimulation (at 12-15 Hz) and from the frontal theta inhibition (half frequency of stimulation from 6-7.5 Hz) in which the awakened frontal lobes also inhibit and calm the motor strip.

Overview Of The ALERT Sessions

Let's take a closer look at the various ALERT sessions, which enables you to practice and master the Sensory Motor Rhythm. There are four groups of sessions, and each one has a specific outcome and purpose. For instance, Group 1 stimulates theta and alpha brainwaves. Group 2 focuses on Sensory Motor Rhythm. Group 3 stimulates beta brainwaves. Group 4 is the final phase which focuses on stabilizing your brainwaves.

ALERT Group 1: Sessions A1 – A4
(Theta and alpha training to dissociate and relax)

These ALERT sessions are designed to help you relax deeply. They will calm impulsiveness, soothe nervous energy and volatile moods, reduce distraction and the tendency to interrupt others.

More specifically, the A1 – A4 sessions use theta-alpha training to reduce fast beta activity in the brain.

Researchers have found that ADHD is a sign of elevated beta activity in the frontal lobes of the brain (Clark, Barry & McCarthy, 2001; Egner, Zech & Grizelier, 2004). A person with an excess in beta activity tends to have poor self-regulation. This makes it difficult to generate the correct brainwave frequency for the task at hand. For instance, you might feel sluggish when you need to get busy and do your work. When this happens, you're parked in the wrong brainwave frequency.

The A1 – A4 sessions correct the problem of poor self-regulation with theta-alpha brainwave training. Researchers have found that theta-alpha training enhances focused attention, creative performance, and working memory tasks (Gevins, Smith, McEvoy & Yu, 1997).

The theta-alpha brainwave training also stimulates the parking or idling frequency of the brain (Swingle, 2008). You may recall that it is important to get in and out of park quickly. Throughout the day, we often transition from one brainwave state to another, and it's important to make the shift quickly and smoothly. Alpha brainwaves play a big part in making these shifts. The speed with which your brain's alpha waves change is an indicator of brain efficiency. When your brain is working at peak efficiency, your reaction time is swift. In other words, you can respond quickly and take action.

What happens when your brain's alpha brainwaves are too slow? Perhaps you've noticed that your reaction time slows down if you're bored, lethargic, overwhelmed, or not paying attention. When the alpha frequencies in the brain slow down, it is difficult to focus, plan and organize, sequence, and follow through on activities (Swingle, 2008).

Excessive frontal alpha in the brain is also related to being overly talkative, fidgety, having restless energy, and sleep difficulties. The good news is that alpha brainwaves can be stabilized with the ALERT. Getting the tempo stabilized also helps your brain to get in and out of park, so that you can make a smooth transition between activities.

Balancing the alpha in the front of the brain is also important to your emotional well-being. If you have too much alpha, you're more likely to be depressed and react negatively to emotional situations. By balancing your alpha brainwaves, you will become more even-keeled and emotionally stable.

Another function of the Group A sessions is to help you be less distracted. The sessions reduce distraction by speeding up theta brainwaves. With ADHD, theta brainwaves tend to be too slow, causing you to daydream and remain in a low arousal state. This also makes it difficult to transition to beta brainwaves, which are needed for focused attention.

When you experience slow theta brainwaves, you will tend to be distracted. Excessive amounts of theta interfere with the ability to concentrate. That is why the ALERT (Group A) sessions aim to speed up slow theta brainwaves.

In the mid-1970s, Dr. Joel Lubar discovered that children suffering from ADHD showed a "dysfunctional brainwave pattern" when examined by electroencephalography (EEG) recording techniques (Lubar & Swartwood, 1995).

The dysfunction was excessive slow theta waves, especially in the central and frontal regions of the brain. Children with ADHD failed to switch from theta to the faster beta brainwaves associated with focused attention. Without constantly changing, high levels of stimulation, ADHD children simply shut down and tune out, producing high theta brainwave activity.

This shortcoming can be corrected with brain training. With the help of the ALERT, slow wave theta EEG activity (4-8 Hz) is speeded up. This is done by increasing faster beta brainwaves in the 14-18 Hz range.

To summarize, the ALERT Group 1 (A 1- 4) sessions use theta-alpha training to (1) reduce fast beta activity (in other words, reduce hyperactivity, impulsivity and distraction), (2) boost alpha brainwaves, which control the parking or idling frequency of the brain (or ability to switch gears and transition between activities), and (3) speed up theta brainwaves, so that it is easier transition to beta brainwaves, which are needed for focused attention.

ALERT Group 2: Sessions A5, A6 & B1
(Training with the SMR for the right hemisphere of the brain)

The ALERT Group 2 sessions use the SMR (12 to 15 Hz) to decrease restlessness, nervous energy, impulsivity, and hyperactivity. This protocol is commonly used to treat ADHD in neurotherapy and other forms of brain training. The Group 2 ALERT sessions build upon the previous sessions (Group 1) and continue to stabilize the faster Beta brainwaves of ADHD. In these sessions, you will practice developing a calm focus and the ability to concentrate without anxiety or urgency.

ALERT Group 3: Sessions B2 & B3 (Training beta brainwaves, 15 to 18 Hz. to improve mood and logical thinking. These sessions focus on the left hemisphere of the brain)

The ALERT Group 3 builds upon the previous session, by continuing to slow down fast beta brainwaves. These sessions will exercise your brain, calm and strengthen it, and increase stability. With these sessions, your brain learns to increase brainwaves that are helpful for improved function. Your mood will become more even-keeled, and you will experience an improved ability to think logically. With regular practice, your brain will also improve its ability to self-regulate. In other words, your brain will learn to automatically decrease excessively fast or slow brainwaves that interfere with good function. Over time, the result is a healthier and better regulated brain.

If you have excessive amounts of certain brainwave frequencies (theta or alpha) in the frontal lobe, you might experience depression or Obsessive Compulsive Disorder (OCD). By training the brain to reduce slower brainwaves and increase faster brainwave activity, these symptoms are often reduced. Over time, new brain behavior is learned and reinforced.

When you give the brain information about itself, it has an enormous capacity for change. The ALERT makes the information available to the brain almost instantly, and asks it to make adjustments. This gives the brain a greater ability to self-manage or regulate.

Another thing that the ALERT does for your brain is that it encourages it to be flexible. Have you ever pulled on a rubber band, and watch it spring back into shape? Life expects us to be like that. We are expected to bounce back after challenges, and keep going. This quality is known as flexibility or resiliency. Like a rubber band, we can train our brain to be flexible, and quickly transition from one brainwave state to another.

Previously, we talked about the parking or idling frequency of the brain. A lack of flexibility (being stuck in a particular state) causes problems, including impulsivity, ADHD, anger, and OCD (Swingle, 2009). Using the ALERT will increase your brainwave state flexibility, as specific regions of the brain are stimulated and activated. Beta frequencies (12 to 20 Hz) are related to brain activation. Training these frequencies can assist in speech, organization, planning, elevating mood, and reducing depression in improved cognitive function and task performance (Swingle, 2009).

Beta brainwave training can also assist in calming the brain, reducing anger, stress-related problems, decreasing over-arousal, improving inhibitory control, and impacting sleep regulation (Swingle, 2009).

ALERT Group 4: Sessions B4 & B5
(Training alpha, beta and SMR to reduce instability)

The Group 4 sessions build upon the previous session by stabilizing the fast beta brainwaves that are typical of ADHD.

When the beta brainwaves are unstable, the brain has difficulty with self-regulation. There are three types of unbalanced beta brainwaves: (1) instability, (2) under-arousal, and (3) over-arousal (Hill & Castro, 2009).

When there is instability, your beta brainwaves have a disorganized or unstable pattern. This means the problem is intermittent. Sometimes, you're on track, and other times it's a struggle to read, listen, and concentrate. The solution for instability is to learn to hold your peak beta brainwaves longer (or stabilize them) in order to condition them into your brain.

When beta brainwaves are under-aroused, you may experience depression and poor attention focus. You may wake up frequently during the night. In this case, beta brainwaves need to be sped up, so they're faster.

Symptoms of over-arousal of beta brainwaves include anxiety, mind chatter, and difficulty falling asleep. In this case, beta brainwaves need to be slowed down. Of course, balance is the key. The ALERT Group 4 sessions will help balance your beta brainwaves as you learn to master the SMR.

The previous ALERT sessions conditioned the left and right hemispheres of the brain separately. Now, these last Group 4 ALERT sessions train the left and right brain hemispheres together, which simultaneously promotes whole brain functioning.

Additional ALERT Sessions

The ALERT C sessions are extra, and can be done after you have listened to each of the previous sessions at least five times each. Here is a little bit of information about these additional sessions.

Session C1: Schumann Resonance

This ALERT session entrains your brain to the earth's predominant natural rhythm, which is the electro-magnetic frequency known as Schumann Resonance. Scientists speculate that the "electro-magnetic chaos" coming from cell phones, microwaves, TVs, and radios interferes with our natural circadian rhythms (Magnetic Therapy Living, 2010; Schumann Resonances, 2010).

This "electro-magnetic chaos" creates anxiety and restless energy, pushes us into Fight or Flight, and boosts stress hormones such as cortisol and adrenaline. The C1 ALERT session is designed to restore natural balance and equilibrium in the mind and body, which may have been aggravated by the man-made electromagnetic signals within the atmosphere.

Did you know that the earth naturally creates electro-magnetic waves which are healthy, calming, and rejuvenating? A German physicist named W. O. Schumann discovered this natural frequency in 1957. While teaching at the Technical University of Munich, Schumann found electromagnetic standing waves in the atmosphere, within the cavity formed by the surface of the earth and the ionosphere. Schumann mathematically calculated that the most predominant electro-magnetic wave occurs at 7.83 Hz. This frequency is known as the Schumann Resonance.

Years later, the Schumann Resonance was used for healing by Dr. Wolfgang Ludwig in Germany, who is known as the Father of Magnetic Therapy. Dr. Ludwig convinced NASA to install Schumann Resonance devices on spacecraft to have a stabilizing effect on the astronauts' health in outer space. When the first astronauts and cosmonauts were out in space, they suffered emotional distress and migraine headaches. Evidently, this happened because they were no longer exposed to the earth's gravity, circadian rhythms, and other natural electro-magnetic waves. Now modern spacecrafts contain a device that simulates the Schumann Resonance (Magnetic Therapy Cure, 2010; Magnetic Therapy Living, 2010; Schumann Resonances, 2010).

Why is the Schumann Resonance beneficial to you and me? Because it helps us to diffuse the electro-magnetic chaos that we are exposed to every day. Consider the electro-magnetic waves that you're exposed to when you use a cell phone, fax machine, listen to the radio in your car, watch TV, or get on the internet. These artificial, man-made electro-magnetic waves drown out the natural signals from the earth. Modern technology is creating an environment that is literally out of tune with nature itself.

Perhaps you've experienced jetlag after a plane trip that involved switching time zones. Or you feel disoriented after riding the subway and then walking through the noisy and crowded city streets. In these cases, you might benefit from entraining to the Schumann Resonance, which creates a state of calm that does wonders for your mind and body. The Schumann Resonance acts as a natural tuning fork for our brainwaves. It induces a specific brainwave frequency that helps your brain let go of stress and restore natural equilibrium.

Session C2: Sensory Motor Rhythm (13.5 to 15 Hz)

This ALERT session further conditions the brain with the SMR (13.5 to 15 Hz.). The C2 session will fine-tune and stabilize the fast beta brainwaves that are typical of ADHD. The C2 session is more progressive than the previous SMR sessions, so it provides the brain with a brisk challenge.

As an option, the C2 ALERT session can be done with the Tru-Vu Omni-screen Eyeset with "view holes". This eyeset is the same as the ALERT eyeglasses, but with view holes cut out so you can see while you're doing a session. These eyesets are popular for athletes to use while exercising, and for students to use while studying or reading. (Additional purchase is required. The ALERT comes with the Tru-Vu Omniscreen Eyeset, but the "view holes" eyeset must be purchased separately. Check the website for details, www.TrainYourBrainTransformYourLife.com).

Session C3: Attention for Children
(Left hemisphere Hz, Right hemisphere 18 & 10 Hz)

This ALERT C3 session was used by school psychologist Michael Joyce (2001) in a clinical study published in the *Journal of Neurotherapy*. In the study, Mr. Joyce provided "light and sound machine" stimulation to 30 children with ADD, and eight children who were reading-challenged.

Mr. Joyce used this specific session, which slows the fast beta frequencies that are typical of ADD. Mr. Joyce measured the ADD children for inattention, impulsiveness, response reaction time, and variability (how inconsistent the child's responses were) using a computerized TOVA continuous performance test. Mr. Joyce observed substantial improvements in attention and reaction time, as well as a reduction in impulsivity and variability. In the reading-challenged group, Mr. Joyce observed an

18-month improvement in instructional reading level, and half-year advancement in grade level.

Session C4: Depression Reduction
(Left hemisphere 10 Hz, Right hemisphere 19 Hz)

This session is recommended for anyone who feels depressed. Using this session balances the alpha brainwaves in the front of the brain, which promotes healthy emotional well-being. Depression may be a sign of a excessive alpha brainwaves. If you have too much alpha, you're more likely to be depressed and react negatively to emotional situations. Like a robust cup of coffee, this session creates a robust alpha response in the brain. As you may recall, a healthy alpha response involves feeling calm and relaxed, but aware of what is happening around you. Alpha represents a state of non-arousal. Like a robust cup of coffee, this session creates a robust alpha response in the brain. As you may recall, a healthy alpha response involves feeling calm and relaxed, but aware of what is happening around you. Alpha represents a state of non-arousal.

Session C5: Brain Brightener
(Recommended for teens, adults and senior citizens)

Try this session if you want to mentally prepare yourself for speaking in front of a group, taking an exam, reading a book, or finishing a project. It will help you to be mentally sharp and ready for new challenges.

The term "brain brightening" was coined by Dr. Tom Budzynski, an American psychologist and Biofeedback pioneer who has conducted many studies on audio-visual stimulation using light and sound machines (Budzynski, 1976; Budzynski, Evans & Abarbanel, 2008).

Dr. Budzynski developed a unique brain training protocol, which combats age-related cognitive decline. Normal aging effects on the brain include less blood flow to the brain, slower metabolism, and slower response times. Budzynski contends that low beta brainwaves need to be aroused (or speeded up) so that your brain can deal with new information, or properly retrieve and apply old information. The Brain Brightener session will boost beta brainwaves, resulting in increased oxygen and blood flow to the brain, faster metabolism, and faster response times.

Session C6: Sound Sync

This session is designed for use with guided imagery, narrative, or music CDs. It is a good session to use with progressive relaxation CDs that help you to relax from head to toe, or a narrative CD that teaches breathing techniques or affirmations. You can use the extra slot in the ALERT, and hook up your CD player to the ALERT. This way, you can listen to your CD with the light and sound stimulation.

●　　●　　●　　●　　●　　●

You've just read an overview of the ALERT sessions, from A to C. With daily practice, you will be able to master the Sensory Motor Rhythm, which has been scientifically proven to help you conquer ADHD. As your brainwave patterns begin to normalize, you will find that many of your non-ADHD symptoms will also improve, such as mood swings, depression, sleep disturbances, temper tantrums, anxiety, and more. You'll love the way the ALERT trains your brain and transforms your life.

Dear Reader,

Do you realize that your brain is plastic? That doesn't mean that your brain is made out of a squishy plastic compound, like silly putty. Brain plasticity refers to the brain's potential to change—which is a tremendous insight into the nature of the brain. Your brain is dynamic—not fixed or wired for life.

Neuroplasticity—the brain's ability to change, grow and develop—may be the most remarkable discovery of the 21st century.

Think of the implications for ADHD. If your brain is capable of change, then ADHD isn't something you have to struggle with for the rest of your life. You can train your brain to strengthen its electro-chemical functioning, and correct any neurotransmitter deficiency or disruption. You can train your brain to master the Sensory Motor Rhythm, so that you will achieve a calm and relaxed focus. You can train your brain to be productive without a sense of urgency or stress. By training your brain, you're also rehabilitating your brain.

Your brain is an organ but it behaves like a muscle. Any part of your brain that is weak or rigid can be trained to be strong, fit and flexible. The more you use your brain, the more you challenge your brain, the stronger it becomes. Using your brain makes it grow and expand. Disuse makes the brain atrophy and weaken.

In this chapter, you will discover:

• Seven things that turn on your brainpower.

• The power of an enriched environment for the brain. When you train your brain, you create an enriched environment for the brain to thrive. Consider the opposite—a boring environment. Boring is bad for the brain. It leads to withdrawal, senility and depression.

• Neuroanatomist Marian Diamond (1999) did experiments with rats in an enriched versus impoverished environment. She found that mental stimulation makes a tremendous difference in the way we think, act and move.

• Three case studies from Norman Doidge's (2007) bestselling book, The Brain That Changes Itself. You'll be inspired by these real life stories of people who trained their brains in order to overcome hardships. Our brain has a remarkable ability to change, even in the most difficult circumstances.

All the best,
Nicky

CHAPTER 14

Your Brain Is Plastic

"You can't teach an old dog new tricks. This proverb says that learning to do new things is difficult because it is hard to forget the old way."
— *Pocket English Idioms*, 2010.

Have you ever watched an old dog take a nap? His body is curled up, and his head is resting comfortably on his paws. The old dog is sleeping so soundly, that you can hear him snoring. Suppose you threw a ball or newspaper and yelled, "Go fetch, boy!" Would the dog be willing to fetch? Probably not. Sometimes, you just can't teach an old dog new tricks.

Some people think this is true about the human brain as well. They assume that you're born with a brain of a certain size and potential, and it's impossible to change your brain's capacity and function. In other words, you can't teach an old dog new tricks. The implication is that your brain can't learn new things (or change, grow and develop) after you reach a certain age. Why? Because your brain is fixed or set in its ways.

In reality, your brain is a growing, changing organ. Your brain is dynamic—not fixed or wired for life. Your brain's capacity and vitality are dependent on how you nourish and treat it. This quality is known as "brain plasticity," or "neuroplasticity." It means that your brain is capable of growing, developing, and changing throughout your life, from birth into old age.

Brain plasticity does not mean that your brain is made out of a squishy plastic compound, like silly putty. Brain plasticity refers to the brain's potential to change—which is a tremendous insight into the nature of the brain.

Think of the implications for ADHD. If your brain is capable of change, then ADHD isn't something you have to struggle with for the rest of your life. You can train your brain to strengthen its electro-chemical functioning. You can train your brain to master the Sensory Motor Rhythm, so that you will achieve a calm and relaxed focus. You can train your brain to be productive without a sense of urgency, anxiety or stress.

By training your brain, you are also rehabilitating your brain. The parts of your brain that are weak or rigid can be trained to be strong, fit, and flexible. You can deliberately stimulate and nudge your brainwaves in the right direction.

This is great news for ADHD—because you're no longer putting a band-aid on a gaping wound. You're rehabilitating your brain. Brain plasticity means that change is possible, and you're responsible for making it happen. When you take Ritalin, drugs are responsible for making you smarter. With brain training, you can take pride in the fact that your brain is doing the work. You're harnessing the natural electricity of your brain. You're training your brain to think faster and smarter. What a difference from taking Ritalin, and being under the influence of drugs. With brain training, you can hold your head high, and take charge of your life.

Critical Period For Brain Plasticity

Let's go back to the old dog. He is still sleeping, that old rascal! Your neighbors want to have some fun, so they bring over their little puppy. The puppy is playfully running around, and yapping loudly. You throw the newspaper, and she fetches it. You toss a ball, and she playfully pushes it back to you.

For years, scientists thought the human brain was like that puppy—growing, developing, and changing. The puppy is able to learn new things, and is up for a challenge. The puppy will grow until she is mature, and then she starts to age. In the same way, the human brain grows until it becomes mature, and then age sets in. Scientists thought the brain was plastic from birth to age 20, and then no more. They believed that the human brain was only capable of change during this critical period.

Within the past 20 years, scientists have examined MRI brain scans and determined that the brain continues to grow and develop well into old age. Of course, it's a different kind of growth from what you experienced in childhood. The brain's circuitry is already in place, and now this system can be fine-tuned, improved or expanded (Brain Fitness Program, 2008; Brain Fitness 2: Sight & Sound, 2009; Brain Fitness Frontiers, 2010).

In infancy and early childhood, the brain undergoes a critical period. It is a special time when your brain is formed and set up. During this time, the brain is organizing and structuring itself. The brain continues to grow and develop until age 20, and then it is fully mature. From this point on, the brain begins to age. However, that does not mean that life is all downhill from there. It does not mean that your best days are behind you. Scientists have discovered that the brain is plastic throughout our lives. Remarkably, the brain can grow, change and develop as we grow older. However, our brain must be stimulated and challenged in order to do so.

You're probably aware of a handful of ways to stimulate and challenge the brain, such as crossword puzzles, learning a foreign language, reading books, or doing something that you have never done before (which requires you to learn a new skill). Actually, there are at least seven things that turn on your brainpower (adapted from Jensen, 2000).

Seven Things That Turn On Your Brainpower

1. **Novelty.** Your brain instantly pays attention when something is out-of-the-ordinary, odd, or new. It's as if your brain says, "Whoa, look at that!" All of a sudden, you have laser-like focus and undivided attention. Your ADHD seems to disappear. Isn't this what happens when children play video games? The brain loves things that are new, unusual ,and different. Novelty or unusual things grab your attention, and turn on your brainpower. Novelty is very good for your brain.

2. **Pleasure.** Your brain loves to feel good. It doesn't have to be a sticky-sweet pleasure either. When you go to an amusement park, you'll notice the variety of ways the park attempts to give you a pleasurable experience. There are adventurous rides. There is a scary, haunted house ride. Sometimes, we like to get scared. Being scared gives you the thrill of danger and suspense. Amusement parks have lots of adrenalin rides, but there is usually a slow-moving train ride—kind of relaxing, with a little bit of a breeze and some scenery. All of these things can make you feel

good, and give you pleasure. In the same way, life offers us a variety of pleasurable experiences that turn on your brain power.

3. **Challenge.** Your brain loves to try new things, and thrives on a challenge. Your brain hates tasks that are too easy or boring. However, something that's too difficult or confusing isn't brain-friendly either. What your brain craves is physical, intellectual, and emotional stimulation. Your brain loves variety and complexity.

4. **Frequency.** The more often you're exposed to something or someone, the more you'll like them. Yes, frequency turns on your brain power. The more often you see someone, the more likely you are to give them your attention and focus. The more frequently that you see someone, the more this person becomes imprinted on your brain.

5. **Feedback.** Your brain loves to experience new things, and get feedback from it. This feedback might be a personal observation, or something you can learn from. For example, suppose you're trying a new gym class and you're sweating and struggling to keep up. You realize that you're getting a good workout, and this is better than sitting home on the couch, watching TV. That's feedback. We need feedback that is specific, consistent, and timely. The brain needs feedback from what ever you're doing, so you can learn. Feedback definitely turns on your brainpower.

6. **Coherence.** When something is coherent (or easy to understand) then it makes sense. Your brain loves to understand people, places, and things. Understanding is a real turn on for your brain. Have you ever looked at something that is disorganized, hard to understand, or confusing—that's a turn off. If something is confusing and you can't get a handle on it quickly, it's as if your brain flips the off-switch and totally loses interest. However, coherence is something that turns your brain on, draws you in, and enables you to pay attention.

7. **Survival.** Your brain is always focused on survival. When you're thirsty, you want something to drink. When you're hungry, you want something to eat. When you're tired, you want to sleep. When you're lonely, you look for companionship. When you're bored and lethargic, you look for an energy boost. All of these things help you to survive. Your brain focuses on your job at work—because you need money to support

yourself and survive. So, when it comes to issues related to survival, your brain is always turned on and paying attention.

Stimulation + Challenge = Brain Boost

When you stimulate and challenge your brain, at least seven positive changes take place inside your head:

1. Brain cells fire and wire, and there are more synapses forming in-between brain cells.

2. Dendrites of the brain grow thicker and denser.

3. Your brain releases neurotransmitters.

4. New neural pathways (or brain maps) are created.

5. There is increased oxygen and blood flow to the brain.

6. Brainwaves are activated, which help you to focus and concentrate.

7. You experience a boost in your arousal level, which helps you to pay attention and focus.

Does Your Brain Really Need Extra Stimulation?

Whenever you stimulate your brain, you boost your ability to listen, read and remember. You might be wondering if your brain needs extra stimulation. Don't we actively use our brains every day? Of course, we do. However, most people often fall into a routine. We often do the same things in the same way. Many behaviors are automatic, such as driving a car. We drive so often that we hardly think about it. We spend time with familiar people, eating familiar foods, and going to familiar places. This does not stimulate and challenge the brain! You are not growing new brain cells this way. Routine activities do not create new neural pathways in the brain. Routine activities cause your brain to become stagnant and bored (Hall, 2001).

"Enriched" Versus "Impoverished" Environment

Neuroanatomist Marian Diamond (1999) wrote about the brain's ability to change in her book, *The Magic Trees of the Mind*. Dr. Diamond conducted experiments with rats and mazes. One group of rats was placed in an "enriched" environment, and the other group was in an "impoverished" environment.

The rats in the enriched environment had lots of toys, spin wheels to run on, balls, levers, sound effects, and food rewards. The impoverished environment was plain and ordinary—just a maze of walls—with no toys or rewards whatsoever.

Dr. Diamond found that rats in the enriched environment found their way through the maze much faster. She also looked at the rat's brains—and found that the rats in the enriched environment had thicker and denser dendrites in the brain. Ultimately, the rats in the enriched environment were mentally healthier and more fit that the impoverished rats.

Dr. Diamond published her findings in her book, *The Magic Trees of the Mind*. The magic trees refers to the dendrites—the branching activity of the neural circuits in the brain.

What does Dr. Diamond's research mean to humans? For one thing, it suggests that mental stimulation makes a tremendous difference in the way we think, act and move.

You see, the enriched environment was mentally stimulating—and this helped the rats to go faster through the maze. The boring, impoverished environment caused poor performance, slow task completion and slow brain growth.

The bottom line is that boredom leads to withdrawal, senility, and depression—whereas enrichment, activity, and challenge promote health and well-being.

Enrichment At Home, School, and Work

We can create an enriched environment at home, school, or work (Jensen, 2000). Enrichment is also used in unexpected places, like amusement parks and zoos. If you've ever visited Walt Disney's Animal Kingdom, you probably remember the Kilimanjaro Safari ride. It is an open-sided safari ride that enables you to see African animals roaming through acres of savanna, rivers, and rocky hills.

If you listen carefully, you'll hear the tour guide talk about enrichment. The tour guide will explain how the Animal Kingdom deliberately creates an enriched environment to keep the animals mentally active, healthy, and happy. For instance, the animal's food is often hidden inside a toy, making it a challenge for the animal to find it and eat it. Another way the animals receive an enriched environment is with the open-air landscape, trees and plants. This enables the animals to roam freely, and enjoy natural surroundings. This is much better then putting the animals in an impoverished cage, or a small room with plain walls that barely gives them enough space to move around. By creating an enriched environment (rather than an impoverished one) the animals live longer, healthier lives.

Enrichment is also a part of the ALERT brain training program. Your brain is stimulated and challenged with pulses of light and sound. It is a rhythm that has been scientifically proven to reduce ADHD, and enables you to train your brain and transform your life.

The Brain That Changes Itself

Neuroplasticity—the brain's ability to change, grow and develop—may be the most remarkable discovery of the 21st century. Canadian psychiatrist Norman Doidge (2007) wrote about it in his bestselling book, *The Brain That Changes Itself: Stories of Personal Triumph From The Frontiers of Brain Science.*

Dr. Doidge shares many case studies of people who overcame hardships by training and conditioning their brains. Here are three case studies from Doidge (2007) which testify to the brain's remarkable power to change.

College professor Dr. Pedro Bach-y-Rita suffered a stroke at age 65. The stroke paralyzed his face and half of his body, leaving him unable to speak. Doctors offered little hope for recovery, and felt it was best to place him in an institution. Even so, his son Dr. Paul Bach-y-Rita (a neurologist) was determined to rehabilitate him. Dr. Paul first taught the professor how to crawl on the ground—a huge task for someone who was half-paralyzed. At the time, the professor needed to be lifted on and off the toilet. Even so, Dr. Paul put knee pads on the professor, and encouraged him to crawl with his weak shoulder and arm supported by a wall. For months, he crawled beside the wall. Next, Dr. Paul brought the professor outside, where he encouraged him to practice crawling in the garden. The neighbors saw this, and said, "This is so disgraceful! Let the old professor rest! He's had a stroke, and needs to rest." Even so, Dr. Paul continued to rehabilitate his father.

Dr. Paul was a medical intern at the time, and didn't have much experience with rehabilitation. His reasoning was that that babies learn to crawl first, and then walk. So that is the approach that he took with his father. They played with marbles and coins on the floor, and encouraged his father to use his weak right hand. They also exercised their hands by scrubbing pots, clockwise and counterclockwise. With lots of practice, the professor eventually learned to crawl, stand on his feet, walk, and speak again. In effect, the professor had retrained his brain to function normally. Three years later, Dr. Pedro Bach-y-Rita returned to teaching college full-time, and eventually fell in love and got married.

Barbara Arrowsmith Young was diagnosed retarded and dyslexic, scoring in the 99th percentile for auditory and visual memory problems. She had trouble pronouncing words, understanding grammar and math concepts, logic, and cause and effect. She also frequently tripped or stumbled. In spite of her difficulties, Ms. Young attended college and graduate school, where she learned about brain plasticity. She began doing mental exercises to re-train her brain. Gradually, Ms. Young's abilities were brought up to the average level with the help of brain training. Today, Ms. Young is no longer considered Learning Disabled. Ms. Young eventually opened up the Arrowsmith School, which offers brain-based assessment to identify weak cognitive functions, as well as brain-training exercises to strengthen these areas.

Cheryl Schilz, age 39, lost her sense of balance after taking the antibiotic Gentamicin. She took the antibiotic for a postoperative infection following a hysterectomy. Unfortunately, the medicine caused Ms. Schilz's internal balance system to malfunction. This caused her head to wobble from side to side. She felt like was perpetually falling, and often staggered as if she were drunk. This problem caused Ms. Schilz to lose her job, and she was forced to live on disability.

Many "wobblers" fall apart emotionally and end up committing suicide. However, Ms. Schilz was treated by Dr. Paul Bach-y-Rita (who was previously mentioned). He introduced Ms. Schilz to a brain training device that would restore her internal balance system. When she wore the device, she stopped wobbling and falling down. The doctors noticed that she was able to hold her balance for 20 seconds after removing the device. It was a "residual effect"—which caused her balance to return to normal, for a brief time. As she continued to use the device, the residual effect lasted longer each time. Her residual effect progressed to hours, to days, and then to four months. Eventually, Ms. Schilz no longer needed to wear the device. In effect, she has trained her brain to restore its natural balance function. Today, Ms. Schilz no longer considers herself a wobbler.

Training The Brain To Overcome Challenges

Isn't it remarkable that these people overcame their problems? They did so by rehabilitating their brains. Their natural cognitive function was restored with various forms of brain training. Their treatment did not involve drugs or surgery. Instead, they used their brain's natural electricity to bring about changes. As they trained their brains, their weak brain functions became stronger and more resilient. The electro-chemical communication in their brain—the wiring and firing— became stronger and more efficient. Any faulty brain wiring was eventually replaced with a new brain map.

Obviously, the brain training these people received is different from the ALERT. The ALERT uses audio-visual brainwave entrainment to help you to conquer ADHD. However, the point of sharing these stories is to show that the brain is capable of physically changing, at any age. It also shows that brain training is worthwhile, and can give you a better quality of life.

The Brain Produces New Neurons

Twenty years ago, scientists believed that the adult brain produced no new neurons. New research indicates the brain does produce new neurons, under certain conditions (Doidge, 2007). What are these conditions? For one thing, you must be in an enriched environment, rather than an impoverished environment. When we become lazy, complacent, and bored, then we are creating an impoverished environment for our brains. When we stimulate and arouse our brains, then we create an enriched environment. The process of creating new brain cells is called "neurogenesis."

Unleash The Powerhouse Inside Your Skull

The forementioned people created new brain cells by unleashing the powerhouse inside their skulls. By training their brains, they also transformed their lives. Isn't that a better solution than medication? What kind of quality of life do people have, if all they can do is swallow pills?

Without brain training, college professor Dr. Pedro Bach-y-Rita would have paralyzed for life. Without brain training, Barbara Arrowsmith Young would continue to be retarded and dyslexic. It is unlikely that she would have launched the Arrowsmith School. Without brain training, Cheryl Schilz would have fallen apart emotionally and probably committed suicide. Just think of the time, money, and heartache that these people were spared.

How about you? Don't let ADHD hold you back. When you train your brain, you will transform your life. My friend, you have within you the ability to accomplish more than you ever have before. Right now, you have the ability within you to exceed all previous levels of accomplishment. You can be and do more than you have ever imagined. All you need to do is learn how and put what you've learned into action.

The Key To Becoming Smarter

Brain training for ADHD is the wave of the future. Instead of drugs, the new trend is rehabilitating the brain to function at a higher level. Brain plasticity is a tremendous breakthrough for ADHD. Because your brain is capable of change, ADHD isn't something that you have to struggle with for the rest of your life. You can rehabilitate your brain. You can train your brain to be fit, flexible, and resilient.

"Exercising your brain is the key to becoming smarter," insists Richard Restak (2002), a renowned neuropsychiatrist and author of *Mozart's Brain And The Fighter Pilot: Unleashing Your Brain's Potential.*

The brain is an organ, but it behaves like a muscle. The more you use your brain, the more you challenge your brain, the stronger it becomes. Using your brain makes it grow and expand. Disuse makes the brain atrophy and weaken. And when you train your brain, you transform your life.

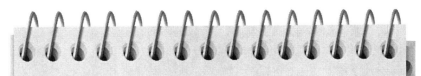

Dear Reader,

So far, we've talked about the ALERT as a brain training device. It's also a relaxation device. Did you know that learning to relax is an important part of conquering your ADHD? It's true. Because being uptight, anxious and stressed makes ADHD worse. Yes, stress actually compounds the problems of distraction, impulsivity, disorganization, and restless energy.

What is stress? It's your body's way of responding to any kind of demand. It is caused by good and bad experiences.

A little stress will sharpen your senses and give you an added push. Too much stress does just the opposite. Too much stress results in exhaustion, confusion, and overwhelm.

Stress is not a big deal, if it's temporary. If that is the case, you could probably go to sleep early, and things will go back to normal. However, stress becomes a problem when it is day after day, with no relief in sight.

Actually, our fast-paced society creates a lot of stress that we can't get away from.

However, we're not powerless over stress. We can do something about it. First of all, we can recognize stress when it strikes. Secondly, we can respond in a calm, level-headed way. We can take a moment to close our eyes, take a deep breath, and whisper a prayer. Take a short break, and allow ourselves a little time to recover from stress. Actually, the best way to deal with stress is to use the adrenaline that your body produces. Get it out of your system. A good cardio workout will release the physical tension from your body. You'll be amazed at how relaxed and energized you feel after a challenging workout.

Another way to release stress is spending 20 minutes in deep relaxation. Just lie down on your bed, put on your ALERT gear, and flip the switch. Aahh, that's instant relaxation! As you relax, you will release tension and anxiety from your mind and body. If your muscles are tense and tight, they will gradually ease up, and become loose, supple, and flexible. The ALERT is an easy and convenient way to calm down and reduce stress.

Stress is like a violin. To make music, the violin strings can't be too tight, or they'll snap. If the strings are too loose, they won't produce sound at all. The right amount of tension lies somewhere in between the two extremes.

All the best,
Nicky

CHAPTER 15

Stress & The Three Rs:
Relaxation, Repair And Rejuvenation

"Do you ever wish for aliens to capture you, so you could escape from your problems?" —Trevor Romain & Elizabeth Verdick (2005), from their book, *Stress Can Really Get On Your Nerves.*

"Stress makes you stupid... or at least it does me. When I'm overwhelmed by deadlines, I say and do some dumb things. I alternately babble or go mute at meetings. I snap at my husband when he calls, and I barely suppress murderous feelings toward tourists who block my path... Even my body becomes unintelligent, refusing to digest food or succumb to sleep." —Lisa Takeuchi Cullen (2007).

"Stupid stress is the same awful feeling as bad stress, but it's about stupid things. Like when I sideswiped my wife's new car in the driveway. Or when our dog wrenched her leg, had surgery, and during her three month recovery period, I pulled a muscle by carrying her all over the house. Stressful, but not tragic. Just stupid.

"Stuff that happens at work is even more stupid. Examples? I've got a million. Anything to do with PowerPoint. When the photocopier goes psycho, especially on Friday afternoon at 4:45 pm. When you spill tomato sauce on your white shirt 15 seconds into the important job interview. When the subway breaks down on your way home from work at 5:45 pm and you must be home by 5:59 pm to take your kid to hockey. Or when you get one of those e-mails, blithely asking you to do something with an air of, 'Surely you can knock this off in 10 minutes,' when you know it will take two days.

"It's not worth fussing about, but you do—because stupid stress is impossible to ignore. Now, what to do about it? Don't smoke, drink, or do that emotional eating thing. Instead, find a way to laugh so hard that you think you're going to pee on yourself." —Paul Fraumeni (2008).

Now that we're both smiling, I wanted to talk to you about a very serious subject. Did you know that stress is the cause of 75 to 80 percent of all visits to a primary care physician? That's according to the American Institute of Stress. People are running to their local pharmacy for stress relief. Americans consume five billion tranquilizers, five billion barbiturates, three billion amphetamines, and sixteen tons of aspirin every year (Colbert, 2008). Much of this medicine is taken to get rid of the headaches, tummy aches, and body pains that are caused by stress.

So far, we've talked about the ALERT as a brain training device. It's also a relaxation device. Learning to relax is an important part of conquering your ADHD. Why? Because being uptight, anxious, and stressed makes ADHD worse. Yes, stress actually compounds the problems of distraction, impulsivity, disorganization, and restless energy.

Stress Versus Relaxed At Work

Suppose you're called into your boss' office. He wants to discuss a project that has gotten off track. Parts of the project are unfinished, mistakes were made, and details need to be corrected. You're worried about being reprimanded, or possibly fired. You're really in a state of distress. You're stressed out. This makes it hard for you to think straight, much less come up with new ideas, or consider a different approach.

Now consider a different scenario. You just finished a big project that you've been working on for months. Feelings of excitement and pride surge through your body. This project couldn't have turned out any better. Your boss calls you into his office, and tells you how pleased he is with your work. He seems to respect you more now. Wow, it doesn't get any better than this! He gives you a high five and you jump up to slap his hand in victory.

In this situation, what is happening to you physically? For one thing, "happy chemicals" are thriving in your brain. You're excited. You've got neural synapses forming, neurotransmitters activating, and there is increased blood flow to the brain. Your "feel good" neurotransmitters, such as serotonin and dopamine, are making positive connections in your brain (Jensen, 2000). You automatically kick into a flow state. Now you can get things done easily and effortlessly. In fact, it doesn't even seem like work. You're just having fun.

When you feel good, doesn't life seem beautiful and sweet? You feel adventurous and optimistic about the future. You're ready to take risks, and maybe even try something new. The sky's the limit now! You're relaxed, easy going, and confident. This kind of state is ideal for getting things done.

Do you see the difference between the two scenarios? Stress has a tremendous impact on your productivity and what you accomplish during the day (Jensen, 2000). If you're calm and relaxed, you're more likely to be productive. That is when your work becomes fun and rewarding. It's like sunshine breaking through the clouds. Your ADHD almost fades away. From head to toe, you're warmed by a confident expectation that you will succeed. There is something about this mindset that fuels you with energy, motivation, and drive. For a person with ADHD, this mindset makes all the difference.

This chapter deals with the dangers of stress, particularly the fight or flight response. Fortunately, there is a way to flip the switch, and turn off stress. With very little effort, you can put the power of relaxation to work for you.

What Is Stress?

Stress is your body's way of responding to any kind of demand. It is caused by good and bad experiences. A little stress will sharpen your senses and give you an added push. Too much stress does just the opposite. Too much stress leaves you feeling exhausted, overwhelmed and confused. It's not a big deal if it's a temporary thing. If that is the case, you could probably go to sleep early, and things will go back to normal. However, stress becomes a problem when it is continuous and on-going, day after day, with no relief in sight.

When you experience stress, there is an immediate change the way you think, look, and feel. There is a tremendous physical change taking place.

Stress Creates Physical Changes In The Body

When you experience stress, your body responds by releasing chemicals into your blood stream, such as adrenaline, cortisol and insulin. It starts with your brain sending signals down your spinal cord to your adrenal glands, telling them to release the hormone adrenaline. Next, adrenaline increases the amount of insulin in your blood.

Your brain's hypothalamus sends signals to your pituitary gland (at the bottom of your brain) telling it to stimulate your adrenal cortex to produce a stress hormone named cortisol. This hormone is very important in your stress response. Cortisol increases your insulin and blood pressure, so that you can escape from danger or defend yourself.

Stress Slows Down Digestion & Metabolism

In a stressful situation, your brain tends to be very practical, and shuts off resources that you don't need. For instance, the part of the brain that is used for critical thinking, judgment, and creativity is short-circuited. Your brain assumes that you don't need these skills right now, because you're getting ready to fight back or run away. To conserve energy, your body also slows down digestion and metabolism. Growth hormones are also switched off, and the immune response is temporarily suppressed.

In the meantime, you breathe faster, so that your body pumps maximum oxygen and energy-rich blood to your muscles. Your liver releases more insulin into your blood, so you are ready for action. Your heart beats faster and faster. Your blood pressure goes up, and your Fight or Flight is now fully activated.

Fight Or Flight Response

The "Fight or Flight Response" was identified in the 1920s by Walter Cannon, a Harvard medical doctor and physiologist. It is a response that is hardwired into your brain to protect you from danger. When stimulated, your brain initiates a sequence of nerve cell firings. Your body releases stress hormones that prepare your body for running away or fighting back. Ideally, your body and mind should return to normal once the stress is over. Do we always go back to normal? Well, we can get stuck in stress mode. Part of the problem is that stress is everywhere.

Stress Is Everywhere

Stress in your mind. You have a long list of things to do, deadlines to meet, and last-minute details to take care of.

Stress in your body. You feel the "wear and tear" of getting older (decreasing eyesight, headaches, sore muscles, and physical pain in your back, chest, arms or legs)

Stress at work or school. You're under the gun of work that demands your time and attention.

Stress at home. You're got bills to pay, cooking, cleaning, laundry, and the challenges of friends and family.

Stress in the car. You must deal with traffic, noise, and weather conditions.

It's no wonder that people feel tied up in knots! We can't think straight or perform at our best. Our fast-paced society creates a lot of stress that we can't get away from. Inevitably, stress is a part of everyday life. Here are ten telltale signs that the pressures of life may be getting a grip on you.

Twelve Signs Of Excessive Stress

1. **Forgetfulness.** Stress short-circuits your memory, at least temporarily. There is so much on your mind that it is hard to think straight.

2. **Irrational thinking.** Under stress, your thinking quickly becomes irrational and confused. Small challenges become huge obstacles.

3. **Feelings of frustration, anger, anxiety, and fear.** Stress can cause our emotions to spiral out of control.

4. **Impulsive behavior.** Stress causes you to say whatever pops into your head, or act on a whim, without thinking about the consequences.

5. **Tendency to make mistakes.** When you're stressed out, it is easy to forget things, leave something behind, or overlook important details.

6. **Headaches, backache, joint or muscle pain.** Stress is stored as tension in the body, which causes physical aches and pains.

7. **Upset stomach, indigestion, heartburn, constipation or diarrhea.** When you experience severe stress, your body releases gastric juices which inflame the throat, stomach, and colon. It's no wonder we have stomachaches and bathroom problems.

8. **Difficulty in falling asleep or waking up.** Stress makes it difficult to wind down and drift off to sleep. Under severe stress, your body continues to pump cortisol, insulin, and adrenaline around the clock, 24-7, even as you sleep. This causes you to awaken groggy and exhausted, rather than well-rested.

9. **Shallow breathing, tightness in the chest, or heart palpitations.** If you feel like an elephant is sitting on your chest, then you're definitely experiencing stress.

10. **Weakened immune system.** Under stress, we are more susceptible to colds, flu, headaches, sore throat, inflammation, and congestion.

11. **Arguments with family and friends.** When stressed, it doesn't take much to fly off the handle, and lose your temper.

12. **Feeling exhausted, run-down & worn out.** When you're dealing with a lot of stress, chemicals like cortisol, insulin, and adrenaline build up in the body, and this overload quickly turns toxic. To compensate, energy is drained from your body, and you feel exhausted and worn out.

Stress Gets Under Your Skin

All of this stress has to go somewhere. Stress is stored as tension in the body. Stress goes deep into your body at the cellular level, and is stored in your muscles and tissues. When stress is stored in the face, it may result in Temporomandibular Joint (TMJ) bruxism (teeth grinding) or migraine headaches. Stress also affects the skeletal system, resulting in back or neck pain (Brown, 2008; Levine, 2000).

Obviously, we need to get rid of the stress. We may not be able to get rid of stress completely, but we can reduce it. We can reduce stress with deep relaxation, exercise, or making a lifestyle change. Otherwise, the stress will continue to build up in the body and cause inflammation.

Think of what happens when you catch a cold. You may experience inflammation in the form of a fever, as your body heats up to eradicate the effects of the invading virus. Suppose you want to get rid of the fever, and swallow some pills. The medicine may reduce the fever, but then the body has to find another way to get rid of the virus. In other words, you're addressing the symptoms, but not the root cause (which is inflammation, caused by stress). Fever can be a good thing. It is the body's way of restoring balance or homeostatis. However, if the inflammation does not return to normal, then it can make you susceptible to arthritus, tendonitus, carpel tunnel syndrome, fibrolylagia, Chronic Fatique Syndrome, Epstein–Barr, Lupus, and other diseases (Brown, 2008; Levine, 2000).

There are serious consequences to chronic stress. The longer that stress lasts, the more the immune system shifts to negative changes. First, you experiences negative changes at the cellular level and later this shifts to broader immune dysfunction. Stress is a problem when it is beyond your control, and there is no relief in sight. That is when stress attacks the immune system, and renders it ineffective. This is the beginning of most diseases (Brown, 2008).

Mind-Body Connection

Initially, Dr. Walter Cannon discovered the Fight or Flight Response in animals. In laboratory experiments, Dr. Cannon noticed that an animal's digestion slowed down dramatically (or even stopped) when animals were anxious, frightened or stressed. This led him to explore the human relationship between emotional states and physiological functioning. As a doctor, Dr. Cannon also spent a lot of time in the emergency room, taking care of patients in distress. Dr. Cannon discovered a mind-body connection. That is, a person's mental and emotional state affects how their body functions. When you are stressed, your emotions stimulate the body's autonomic nervous system. As mentioned previously, this leads to many changes in your muscles, glands and body functions such as increased secretion of adrenaline, increased heart rate, blood pressure, perspiration, and decreased digestion. Today, these changes are all well known symptoms of what can be called a stress response.

Is Stress Ever Good For You?

Yes, stress is good for the body in small doses. Cortisol improves your memory, and enables you to recall names, addresses, and phone numbers. Adrenaline gives you energy and strengthens your immune system. If your life is in danger, adrenaline gives you a burst of energy to run away faster or fight harder. It's exactly what you need if your life is in danger. The stress gives you some extra energy to take off running or defend yourself.

But what it you're not in danger? Suppose you're in a stressful situation, and your boss, co-worker, or spouse is yelling at you. Your adrenaline levels are high. Maybe you'd like to punch them in the face, or take off running. Of course, that wouldn't solve anything, would it? Responding like that is counterproductive, so you'd probably pull yourself together, and swallow or stuff your feelings.

Regrettably, that is not a healthy response either. When we swallow or stuff our feelings, we tend to deny our emotions, rather than deal with them. This denial causes us to feel resentful, angry, sorry for ourselves, depressed, worn-out, overwhelmed, tense, or anxious.

When we repeatedly respond to stress this way, the mechanism that is meant to save your life becomes overused (Jensen, 2000). The stress starts to build up, and has no place to go. Prolonged distress (or being constantly on-guard) will wear you down, and has a toxic effect on your body. It impairs your ability to think clearly.

When stress has no place to go, the hormones build up in our body and become toxic. Cortisol builds up and causes brain cells to shrink.

We become jittery, anxious, and forgetful. Unused adrenaline makes us depressed and lethargic. There is less oxygen going to our brain, heart, and other vital organs. Left untreated, stress makes us vulnerable to high blood pressure, possible stroke/heart problems, flus and colds, tense muscles, backache, and mental breakdown.

If Stress Is The Problem, What's The Solution?

Stress makes us feel overwhelmed, restless, distracted and disorganized. However, the good news is that we are not powerless over stress. We can do something about it.

First of all, we can recognize stress when it strikes. Secondly, we can respond in a calm, level-headed way. We can take a moment to close our eyes, take a deep breath, and whisper a prayer. Take a short break, and allow ourselves a little time to recover from stress.

Actually, the best way to deal with stress is to use the adrenaline that your body produces. Get it out of your system. A good cardio workout will release the physical tension from your body. For example, try bicycling, running on a treadmill, jogging, step aerobics, Zumba, or a group fitness class. You'll be amazed at how relaxed and energized you feel after a challenging workout.

Another way to release stress is spending 20 minutes in deep relaxation. Just lay down on your bed, put on your ALERT gear, close your eyes, and flip the switch. Aahh, that's instant relaxation. As you relax, you release tension and anxiety from your mind and body. If your muscles are tense and tight, they will gradually ease up, and become loose, supple, and flexible. The ALERT is an easy and convenient way to calm down and reduce stress.

I hope this chapter has increased your awareness of stress, and it's effect on the mind and body. Stress is like a violin. To make music, the violin strings can't be too tight, or they'll snap. If the strings are too loose, they won't produce sound at all. The right amount of tension lies somewhere in between the two extremes. Somewhere in-between good stress and bad stress is your creative genius. This is the key to surviving and thriving in a fast-paced world.

Dear Reader,

When you relax deeply, you turn off the stress response. Stress never goes away completely, but we can reduce stress (and keep it under control) by learning to relax and let go.

With ADHD, we tend to be sensitive to the pressures of life. We don't always know how to handle conflict, get organized, or manage our time. If we feel overwhelmed, it is difficult to focus and get things done. Plus, there is the added pressure of tasks that are boring. Do you ever find yourself "stuck"-- no motivation when you have work to do? That's when you need an extra burst of energy to pull yourself together. You need to get on task and finish the work that you've started.

Actually,, it's a good time to use the ALERT. Taking a 22-minute catnap with the ALERT will reduce stress, restore, and rejuvenate you. It is a quick and easy way to get a grip on your ADHD, and take charge of your day.

When you're relaxing with the ALERT, your body enters into a regenerative state. As you breathe deeply, there is more oxygen and blood going to your heart, lungs and skin. Your breathing and heart rates slow down to a comfortable pace.

(Continued)

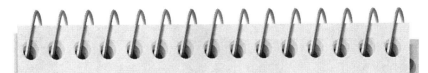

As you relax, there is a tremendous sense of physical release. Your blood pressure decreases. Your mind chatter becomes quiet, and feelings of anger and frustration are released. A wonderful burst of energy comes as you relax and let go.

When you relax deeply, your body flips a switch that gradually restores balance. Scientifically, the process is known as "homeostasis." As you relax, you will let go of the tension and anxiety. Your body makes adjustments in order to normalize, or create a balanced and stable environment inside your body. That is why relaxation is the perfect antidote for stress.

Ultimately, the ALERT frees your brain and body to function as they are created to be. Your natural state is calm, relaxed, and easy going. It is the way you feel in the morning, as you wake up in a warm, comfy bed. It is a relaxed, comfortable and energized feeling. It's top-of-the-morning energy.

Your brain is one of the most active organs your the body, and it requires uninterrupted energy. Relaxation is like fuel for the brain.

All the best,
Nicky

CHAPTER 16

The Three Rs:
Relaxation, Rejuvenation And Restoration

"It might surprise you that a lot of stress enters through your eyes. Bright sun or car headlights make you squint. Clashing colors can make you irritable. Sudden movements make you flinch. Wind and dust make your eyes water and blink. Long hours reading make your eyes sore. Fast-paced commercials can exhaust your eyes. The brash ads on signs, billboards, and magazine ads are all brightly competing to grab your attention and hold it. We've created a frenetic modern visual environment that is a continuous assault on eyes that evolved to scan peaceful green and gold savannahs.

"There are also emotional stressors that involve the eyes. Urban clutter or household mess— the visual equivalent of noise— can wear you down. Overwork can not only tire your eyes but make you sick of looking at your papers. Some days, everywhere you look you see reminders of jobs undone, hopes dashed, obligations unfulfilled, opportunities lost, defeats suffered.

"Your eyes are pointed outward because they are your primary tool for observing and comprehending the external world. Your eyes are literally your lookouts, constantly scanning the horizon for approaching danger or opportunity.

"Tired eyes seek blackness as a rest from vigilance and the daily image assault. Blackness shuts you off from the real world and forces you to look in on yourself— a physical impossibility and a spiritual necessity.

"Try enjoying blackness a couple of times a day. It just takes a minute. Seated at a desk or table, put the heels of your palm directly over your closed eyes. Block out all light without putting too much pressure on your eyelids.

"Try to see the color black. You may see other colors, or images, but focus on the color black. Use a mental image to remember the color black: Black cats, black holes in space, the back of a dark closet.

"Tell yourself that you don't have to look at anything right now. Let the muscles around your eyes relax— your eyelids, under your eyes, the crease between your brows, your forehead, your cheeks.

"After a minute, slowly lower your hands and gently open your eyes. Remind yourself throughout the day that at almost any moment you can close your eyes and escape into blackness." —Matthew McKay & Patrick Fanning (1997), *The Little Book of Relaxation and Stress Reduction*, p. 47-49.

When you think about relaxation, what comes to mind? Perhaps a warm bath, quietly watching TV, reading a book, or enjoying dinner with family or friends. These activities are relaxing, but don't always provide the deep release of tension that your body craves. With the ALERT, you will experience a state of deep relaxation, almost like a massage. The audio-visual rhythm is specifically designed to help you to let go physical tension in your body, and neutralize feelings of anxiety, fear, and overwhelm.

When you're relaxing with the ALERT, your body enters into a regenerative state. As you breathe deeply, there is more oxygen and blood going to your heart, lungs and skin. Your breathing and heart rate slows down to a comfortable pace. Your blood pressure decreases. There is a tremendous sense of physical release. Your mind chatter becomes quiet, and feelings of anger and frustration are released. A wonderful burst of energy comes as you relax and let go.

When you relax deeply like this, you are experiencing the "rest and digest" response. As you rest and digest, your nerves become calm, and your body gradually returns to its regular function.

It's the opposite of the Fight or Flight Response. With Fight of Flight, your brain turns off resources it doesn't need: Digestion, immune response, and also the part of your brain that is used for critical thinking, judgment, and creativity. Miraculously, all of these things come back when you rest and digest. Your gastro-intestinal tract is now able to metabolize the food you've eaten, so your body can break it down and convert it to energy. Rest and Digest also activates peristalsis, those wave-like contractions that enable you to have a bowel movement.

What Happens When You Relax

When you relax deeply, your body flips a switch that gradually brings you back into equilibrium. Scientifically, the process is known as "homeostasis." As you relax, you let go of the tension and anxiety. Your body makes adjustments in order to normalize, or create a balanced and stable environment inside your body. That is why relaxation is the perfect antidote for stress.

Medical doctor Walter Cannon (1932) coined the term homeostasis, in his book *The Wisdom Of The Body.* Dr. Canon claims there is an innate intelligence in the body, which is constantly striving towards internal balance. Very simply, homeostasis means that your body is always working to create a stable and balanced environment on the inside, in order to keep you alive and healthy.

Consider what happens when you exercise. As you work out, you begin to feel hot and sweaty. As sweat evaporates from the surface of your skin, you cool down. In this way, sweating lowers your body temperature and brings it back to normal. That's the power of homeostasis at work.

Other Examples Of Homeostasis:

- Your blood clots when you bleed
- Your body repairs and regenerates damaged tissues
- Your body maintains fluid and electrolyte balance
- Your body maintains blood sugar levels
- Your body maintains a proper acid-ph balance in your blood & kidneys
- Your immune system responds to bacteria and viruses
- Your body temperature is maintained within a normal range

When you relax deeply, you turn off the stress response. There will always be stress in our lives. It never goes away completely, but we can reduce stress (and keep it under control) by learning to relax and let go.

Relaxation Gives You An Energy Boost

With ADHD, we tend to be sensitive to the pressures of life. We don't always know how to handle conflict, get organized, or manage our time. If we feel overwhelmed, it is difficult to focus and get things done. Plus, there is the added pressure of tasks that are boring. That's when we need an extra burst of energy to pull ourselves together. We need to get on task and finish the work that we've started.

Actually, it's a good time to use the ALERT. Taking a 22-minute catnap with the ALERT will reduce stress, restore, and rejuvenate you. It is a quick and easy way to get a grip on your ADHD, so you can take charge of your day.

You may recall from chapter one that I described my personal experience with the ALERT. The benefits that I've experienced include energizing my brain to read, study or solve problems; boosting my mood, helping me to calm down, relaxing and stabilizing my emotions; and reducing stress and anxiety. All of these things help me to be more productive with my work. In the back of this book, there are more testimonies from ALERT users who have experienced similar results.

The beautiful thing about deep relaxation is that you can reap the results while lying flat on your back, with your eyes closed. The more you train your brain to relax, the more this becomes an automatic response. Your brain's neural pathways that are activated with relaxation will become deeper and stronger. In time, your mind will actually prefer relaxation to stress.

Chilling Out With The ALERT

When you relax, you set aside three activities which would normally take up most of your mental resources: Vision, muscle activity and internal dialogue (Baker, 2001).

1. **Vision.** When you close your eyes, everything fades to black. You are quieting your brain's expenditure on three-dimensional color vision. About 60 percent of your body's resources are spent on making a 3D color picture of the world around you. When you close your eyes, your brain no longer needs to hold on to that 3D color image. As you let go, you release

the mental processing and emotions that go along with it. When you turn off your vision, you instantly release tension from your mind and body.

2. **Muscle activity.** As you focus your eyes on the printed words of this page, you are using your eye muscles. Of course, you have muscles all over your body, from head to toe. You might be surprised how much muscle activity is involved in sitting at your desk and reading this book. You engage your muscles throughout the day, which takes effort and energy. When you are lying down and relaxing with the ALERT, you temporarily suspend the muscle activity of your body. You will find this extraordinarily refreshing, as your body resynchronizes the rhythms that have gotten out of harmony in the fast pace of the day.

3. **Internal dialogue.** There is a voice inside your head that talks to you. Most of the time, you are in control of this voice, your inner dialogue. However, the cares of the day can fill your mind with worry, doubt, and fear. Stress and the responsibilities of the day can cause your mind chatter nonstop.

"The best way to stop mind chatter is to keep the language center of your brain busy without letting it engage in thinking," suggests Dr. Sidney McDonald Baker (2001), in his book *The Circadian Prescription*. Does that sound impossible? It's exactly what happens when you relax deeply with the ALERT.

When you use the ALERT, your internal dialogue gradually slows down and becomes quiet. You no longer need to think about anything. As you let your thoughts go, you will enter a state of relaxation unlike anything you have ever experienced. This enables the brain's natural energy to be restored.

When you stop the chattering mind, if only for a few minutes, you energize your brain cells. You clear out the static and tune into a natural state of calm. Simply relaxing and letting go will restore energy levels and rejuvenate you.

It's nice to relax deeply with our eyes closed, but will it make a difference in everyday life? After all, we spent most of the day with our eyes wide open. What happens when we relax deeply? Is relaxation something temporary, which only lasts while we close our eyes, or does it make a difference in everyday life?

This is why researching and writing this book is so meaningful for me. It has caused me to realize how deep relaxation can reduce stress, and actually creates physiological changes in the body. Yes, these changes are temporary, but the more we practice them, the more it becomes a conditioned, automatic response. We can condition ourselves to let go of stress, and activate the Rest and Digest Response. As a quick review, here are at least nineteen things that deep relaxation does for your body:

Nineteen Things That Deep Relaxation Does For Your Body

1. Suspends vision, muscle activity and internal dialogue
2. Slows your heart rate
3. Lowers blood pressure
4. Slows down your breathing rate
5. Increases oxygen & blood flow to major muscles & brain
6. Reduces muscle tension in the body
7. Lowers stress hormones in the blood (cortisol, adrenaline & insulin)
8. Activates the Rest and Digest Response
9. Stimulates neural cells in the brain, resulting in growth and change
10. Reduces anger and frustration
11. Improves focus, concentration, memorization and retention
12. Boosts energy levels
13. Reduces hyperactivity and restlessness
14. Increases the power of the immune system to eliminate toxins
15. Boosts resistance to infection
16. Eliminates (or greatly reduces) chronic depression and anxiety
17. Normalizes sleep patterns (falling asleep and waking up)
18. Helps to create an energized, peak performance state
19. Eliminates or reduces chronic and transient pain

Awakening The Sleeping Giant

When you use the ALERT regularly, you will cultivate the Relaxation Response. It is a state of deep rest that changes your physical and emotional responses to stress. As we mentioned earlier, it is the opposite of the Fight or Flight Response. The Relaxation Response activates "rest and digest" and the other benefits previously mentioned. It is the perfect way to bring what you learn behind closed eyes into open-eyed, everyday living.

Many contemporary medical doctors have written about the Relaxation Response, such as Harvard cardiologist Herbert Benson, Dr. Bernie Siegel, Dr. Andrew Weil, and Dr. Carl O. Simonton—just to name a few.

The Relaxation Response offers something that isn't found in a pill or capsule. You already have it inside of you. It's a sleeping giant that needs to be awakened. As you relax deeply, you awaken your innate intelligence to create a balanced and stable environment inside your body. It's the power of homeostasis that brings your mind and body into equilibrium. Truly, this is a miracle! Something miraculous happens when you tap into your body's natural ability to restore and rejuvenate itself.

As you learn to relax, your awareness will also increase. You will become more aware of muscle tension and other physical sensations of stress. Once you know what the stress response feels like, you can make a conscious effort to relax the moment you start to feel stressed. This can prevent stress from spiraling out of control.

Over time, the ALERT will also give you a higher threshold for stress. Instead of responding to stressful situations with anger, frustration, and anxiety, you will learn to respond in a calm and levelheaded way. You can let go of negative emotions that hold you back from being all you can be.

Ultimately, the ALERT frees your brain and body to function as they are created to be. Your natural state is calm, relaxed, and easy going. It is the way you feel in the morning, as you wake up in a warm, comfy bed. It is a relaxed, comfortable, and energized feeling. It's top-of-the-morning energy. Your brain is one of the most active organs your the body, and it requires uninterrupted energy. Relaxation is like fuel for the brain.

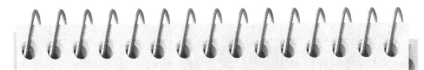

Dear Reader,

In this final chapter, you'll find a recap of the five ADHD challenges, and how the ALERT works to fix them. I hope this book has given you the courage to say no to Ritalin, and yes to brain training.

You might be wondering, "If I use the ALERT for 60 days, will my ADHD disappear forever, and never come back?"

Unfortunately, there is always the possibility of relapse. Any major life change can trigger your ADHD: Losing your job, ending a relationship, being in a car accident, a bitter argument, death of a loved one, etc.

Even positive changes can trigger your ADHD, such as getting married, starting a new job, or moving into a new house.

If your brainwaves become unbalanced for any reason, they might not return to normal after the event has passed. If this happens, it's time for an ALERT maintenance session. Be sure to use the ALERT every day until your ADHD improves.

Boredom is another landmine for ADHD. If we don't get enough stimulation, then we're bored.

(Continued)

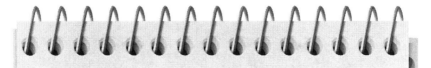

Unfortunately, there will always be boring people, places, and events that trigger our ADHD.

We'll meet people that will drive us crazy, take forever to get to the point, or drag their feet. There will be tasks and assignments that we hate doing, books that are hard to understand, and unpleasant situations that make us want to throw up our hands in defeat. Let's face it, if something is boring, it's very difficult to do. The temptation to disengage and be distracted is always there.

Fortunately, you have a secret weapon in your arsenal. The ALERT is a handy tool that you can use anytime, anyplace. It will boost your arousal, so that you can focus and pay attention. It calms your restless energy, and gives you the stimulation that you desperately crave. It boosts the neurotransmitters in your brain, so that you can think clearly and get organized. It speeds up sluggish ADHD brainwaves, so that you're in the right frame of mind. Now you can be prepared for whatever comes your way, good or bad. When you train your brain, you also transform your life.

All the best,
Nicky

P.S. Thanks for reading these letters! ☺

CHAPTER 17

Five Challenges, Five Solutions For ADHD

"When the brain is restored to its proper functioning, it allows the achievement of all its intrinsic abilities. Brains are exquisitely designed to pay attention and to comprehend information; to achieve full human potential; to focus, think, reason, dream, and create." — Robert Hill & Eduardo Castro (2002), *Getting Rid Of Ritalin.*

Finally, we've reached the last chapter of this book. We've covered a lot of territory in these pages. I commend you for sticking with it, and not giving up until you reached the end. I hope this book has given you the courage to say no to Ritalin, and yes to brain training. As a quick review, here are five ADHD challenges, and how the ALERT works to correct them.

 # 1. Challenge: ADHD is a sign of weak electro-chemical communication between brain cells. Your brain cells misfire and miswire, or there aren't enough neurotransmitters for the signal to go through. This short-circuits your brain cells' ability to talk to each other. It causes distraction, poor focus and concentration, and difficulty getting organized.

Solution: The ALERT uses audio-visual stimulation to ramp up your brain's natural electricity, and condition your brain for peak performance. The stimulation that you receive from the ALERT encourages your brain cells to wire and fire correctly, produce a stable supply of neurotransmitters, and successfully connect to the neighboring neurons at the synapse.

 # 2. Challenge: People with ADHD have sleepy brains, or low arousal. That's why it's pure torture to listen to a boring lecture or wait in line. Boring activities don't challenge, stimulate, or arouse our brain. We crave stimulation, and when we don't get it, we find ourselves distracted and disengaged.

Solution: Low arousal is linked to low dopamine levels in the brain, as well as an underactive prefrontal cortex (Gray & Amen, 2003). This causes you to feel bored, tired, restless, hyperactive, impulsive, and disruptive. Brain training with the ALERT naturally boosts your dopamine levels using the Sensory Motor Rhythm. The ALERT does this with gentle light and sound stimulation to the visual cortex and auditory cortex. As a result, your brain naturally compensates for any neurotransmitter deficiency that it may be experiencing due to ADHD. As dopamine levels become stable, your prefrontal cortex becomes more active (Monastra, 2005). The ALERT also increases oxygen and blood flow to the brain. This gives you a extra boost in arousal, so you can think fast on your feet.

 # 3. Challenge: Having ADHD is like being rhythmically challenged. You're out of step with the rhythm of focusing, concentrating, remembering, and getting organized.

Solution: The sights and sounds of the ALERT will train your brain for peak performance. Using the ALERT enables you to practice and master the Sensory Motor Rhythm, which has been clinically proven to reduce ADHD by helping you achieve a relaxed focus, improved concentration, and the ability to tune out distractions. Mastering this rhythm soothes restless energy, quiets impulsivity, and minimizes distractions.

 # 4 Challenge: It's very hard to get rid of ADHD because your brainwaves are parked in the wrong place. Your brainwaves are stuck in an ADHD pattern, and will not return to a healthy balance on their own. In fact, your brain interprets ADHD as normal, and works to maintain it. With ADHD, the power of homeostasis works against you.

Solution: With the ALERT, the Sensory Motor Rhythm interrupts your regularly scheduled ADHD program with a very important message, "Come dance with me!" Yes, you've been doing the ADHD jive for years, but this new Sensory Motor Rhythm is fun, and your brain likes it. Your brain starts to dance along with the rhythm, and something magical happens. Your brainwaves are gently nudged in the direction of healthy balance. Gradually, your brainwaves are fine-tuned and stabilized. Your brain begins to changes electro-chemically. Eventually, your brain creates a new brain map, and the old ADHD map is no longer used.

 # 5. Challenge: Stress makes ADHD worse. It causes your brain to work less when you need it most. Stress causes irrational thinking, overwhelm, impulsive behavior, and the tendency to make mistakes.

Solution: The ALERT enables you to relax deeply, so that you can let go of stress. You can turn off the Fight or Flight response, and activate the Rest and Digest response. Relaxation is like fuel for the brain. It restores, regenerates, and rejuvenates you.

That's the five challenges of ADHD and the five solutions provided by the ALERT. Now you're ready to train your brain and transform your life!

One thing that I haven't said much about is oxygen. The ALERT increases the amount of oxygen going to your brain. Oxygen is the fuel for all brain activities that lead to high thinking. It's important because a stable supply of oxygen helps you to think fast on your feet. In fact, oxygen is something that your brain desperately needs to survive. Your brain uses approximately 20% of your body's total oxygen consumption. That is a hefty amount of oxygen, when you consider that the brain only takes up two percent of your whole body mass. Whenever your oxygen intake goes down, you will feel sleepy and lethargic. This is the main reason why we feel sleepy after big meals. Our digestive system uses up large amounts of oxygen to digest the food that we have eaten (Patel, 2010 & Altman, 2007).

The ALERT also increases blood flow to the brain. Your blood cells carry oxygen to your brain and the rest of your organs. The brain accounts for more than 25 percent of the body's blood flow. Without adequate blood flow, your brain is deprived of oxygen and thus is unable to operate at peak efficiency (Amen, 2010; Patel, 2010; Altman, 2007).

Your brain's energy, as well as the energy in the rest of your body, is made by energy powerhouses called mitochondria that are found in each cell. Oxygen enables the mitochondria in your brain cells to pump out an energy chemical called Adenosine Triphosphate, or ATP. Without adequate levels of ATP, your brain is drained of energy and its function decreases (Sears, 2003).

As you age, there is decreased blood flow to the brain and the mitochondria become less efficient at pumping out ATP. Without adequate blood flow, your brain is deprived of oxygen and thus is unable to manufacture enough ATP to operate at peak efficiency. Below a critical level of ATP production, brain cells can begin to die. This is what happens with a stroke. The victim's blood flow and oxygen to their brain is restricted, and brain cells in that region die (Sears, 2007). The bottom line is that the increased oxygen and blood flow from using the ALERT is good preventative care for your brain.

As the title of this book claims, you can conquer ADHD in 60 days, without Ritalin. Doctors commonly prescribe Ritalin (and other stimulant medication) for ADHD, but it's not an effective long-term solution. On the positive side, Ritalin boosts neurotransmitters, speeds up slow brainwaves, and increases arousal in the brain. However, long term use of Ritalin negates these benefits and makes ADHD worse. Having ADHD is like sitting on a tack. You could take medicine for relief, but it's best to simply pull out the tack. When you train your brain with the ALERT, you accomplish the same thing as Ritalin, without the side effects. Plus, brain training makes more permanent and lasting changes in the brain.

You might be wondering, "If I use the ALERT for 60 days, will my ADHD disappear forever, and never come back?" The answer to that question is yes and no. Yes, the ALERT will help you to conquer ADHD, but there is always the possibility of relapse. The ALERT gives you a new brain map for learning. It creates new neural pathways, and the old ADHD map is no longer used. These changes are permanent, and yours to keep. The only thing that may cause you to regress is trauma or crisis. This could be anything: Losing your job, ending a relationship, being in a car accident, a bitter argument, death of a loved one, etc.

Even positive changes can trigger your ADHD, such as getting married, starting a new job, or moving into a new house. Unfortunately, your brainwaves can become unbalanced for any reason, and might not return to normal after the event has passed. If this happens, it's time for an ALERT maintenance session. Be sure to use the ALERT every day until your ADHD improves.

Boredom is another landmine for ADHD. If we don't get enough stimulation, we're bored. And there will always be boring people, places, and events that trigger our ADHD. We'll continue to meet people that drive us crazy, take forever to get to the point, and drag their feet. There will be tasks and assignments that we hate doing, books that are hard to understand, and unpleasant situations that make us want to throw up our hands in defeat.

Let's face it, if something is boring, it's very difficult to do. The temptation to disengage and be distracted is always there. Fortunately, you have a secret weapon in your arsenal. The ALERT is a handy tool that you can use anytime, anyplace. It will boost your arousal, so that you can focus and pay attention. It calms your restless energy, and gives you the stimulation that you desperately crave. It boosts neurotransmitters in your brain, so that you can think clearly and get organized. It speeds up sluggish ADHD brainwaves, so that you're in the right frame of mind. Now you can be prepared for whatever comes your way, good or bad.

There will always be ADHD triggers, but now you can manage your symptoms and keep things under control. The more you practice the Sensory Motor Rhythm, the more this rhythm becomes a conditioned, automatic response. This doesn't mean you'll turn into a robot. The ALERT won't make you think or act in a mechanical or submissive way. It's not mind control. Instead, the ALERT sets you free from ADHD symptoms that hold you back from being all you can be. It's those pesky symptoms like restless energy, stress, distractibility, impulsivity, and poor concentration. These things can keep you from being productive and making your dreams a reality. With the ALERT, you can manage your ADHD symptoms, so that the real you shines through.

Hopefully, we've learning something from our ADHD. We're learning how to respond to life in an empowering rather than a disempowering way. Instead of responding with anger, frustration and hopelessness, we can talk to ourselves in an empowering way. We can make our self-talk upbeat and positive, rather than sarcastic, cruel or demeaning. Whenever we're stressed out, we can also cultivate the Relaxation Response, and awaken our innate intelligence to create a stable and balanced environment in our mind and body.

Remember the stray cats from Dr. Sterman's lab experiment? They were exposed to the toxic rocket fuel, yet they were immune to it, because they were trained with the Sensory Motor Rhythm. You can be like that.

By using the ALERT, you can be stronger and more resilient, bouncing back from crisis. You can also develop a higher threshold for stress, and respond to it in a calm and level-headed way.

Have your ever experienced a dry spell? In my backyard, the sun had taken it's toil on the grass. Parts of the grass were brown and withered. I wondered if there was any life left in that soil. I got out my garden hose, and watered the lawn. That's when a funny thing happened. The ground initially resisted the water! Here the soil is parched dry and desperately needs water. But the water beads up, almost as like drops of oil. I shook my head, and whispered: "Come on, dry soil, drink up that water!"

Silly me, thinking that this stubborn soil would respond to my words. But, as I put the hose away, something amazing happened. The water slowly absorbed into the ground. Yes, the soil's resistance had given way. The soil drank in the moisture that it needed.

Having ADHD is like experiencing an emotional drought. Something inside of us hungers and thirsts for more than our present circumstances. We crave stimulation and arousal. We need it like dry ground needs water. We look for ways to flip the switch and turn on our brainpower. We struggle to be in the right frame of mind.

Fortunately, the ALERT can rescue us from ADHD. It rhythmically stimulates and soothes our restless energy. It quenches our thirst for stimulation. It relaxes, restores and rejuvenates us. Occasionally, there will be times that we buckle and resist the changes that are taking place. We might remember painful or embarrassing things from our past, and wrestle with those feelings. However, if we can just let go and relax, the fear and anxiety will fade away. Like water seeping into the dry ground, these intense feelings will disappear. My friend, if you're ready for that, then you can train your brain and transform your life.

Five-Day Method
For The ALERT 60-Day Brain Training Program

Instructions: This program is for 60 consecutive days. Do a session for five days and then go on to the next session. If you miss a day, pick up where you left off. If you miss more than one day, please start over at session A-1. You need consistency for the ALERT to be effective.

If you feel like five days is not enough time, you could do each session for seven days before going on to the next session. (In this manner, it will take you longer to complete the program, but this gives you more time to practice and master the sessions).

For each day that you do an ALERT session, fill in the circle. The numbers 0 to 6 after the circle is for recording your "relaxation landmark" after the session. Just circle the number that best describes your session. This will help you to be more aware of your progress. Ultimately, the goal is to have a landmark of six during your sessions. It will take some time to reach this landmark, but you should be able to reach it by the end of 60 days, if not sooner. (For a detailed description of the relaxation landmarks, see chapter 4).

Week 1: Session A-1 (Theta-Alpha training to dissociate and relax).
Day 1   O   0 1 2 3 4 5 6
Day 2   O   0 1 2 3 4 5 6
Day 3   O   0 1 2 3 4 5 6
Day 4   O   0 1 2 3 4 5 6
Day 5   O   0 1 2 3 4 5 6

Week 2: Session A-2 (Theta-Alpha training to dissociate and relax).
Day 1   O   0 1 2 3 4 5 6
Day 2   O   0 1 2 3 4 5 6
Day 3   O   0 1 2 3 4 5 6

Day 4   O 0 1 2 3 4 5 6
Day 5   O 0 1 2 3 4 5 6

Week 3: Session A-3 (Theta-Alpha training to dissociate and relax).
Day 1   O 0 1 2 3 4 5 6
Day 2   O 0 1 2 3 4 5 6
Day 3   O 0 1 2 3 4 5 6
Day 4   O 0 1 2 3 4 5 6
Day 5   O 0 1 2 3 4 5 6

Week 4: Session A-4 (Theta-Alpha training to dissociate and relax).
Day 1   O 0 1 2 3 4 5 6
Day 2   O 0 1 2 3 4 5 6
Day 3   O 0 1 2 3 4 5 6
Day 4   O 0 1 2 3 4 5 6
Day 5   O 0 1 2 3 4 5 6

Week 5: Session A-5 (Training with the SMR, part 1)
Day 1   O 0 1 2 3 4 5 6
Day 2   O 0 1 2 3 4 5 6
Day 3   O 0 1 2 3 4 5 6
Day 4   O 0 1 2 3 4 5 6
Day 5   O 0 1 2 3 4 5 6

Week 6: Session A-6 (Training with the SMR, part 2).
Day 1   O 0 1 2 3 4 5 6
Day 2   O 0 1 2 3 4 5 6
Day 3   O 0 1 2 3 4 5 6
Day 4   O 0 1 2 3 4 5 6
Day 5   O 0 1 2 3 4 5 6

Week 7: Session B-1 (Training with the SMR, part 3).
Day 1   O 0 1 2 3 4 5 6
Day 2   O 0 1 2 3 4 5 6
Day 3   O 0 1 2 3 4 5 6
Day 4   O 0 1 2 3 4 5 6
Day 5   O 0 1 2 3 4 5 6

Week 8: Session B-2 (Training with beta, 15 – 18 Hz to improve mood and logical thinking, left hemisphere of the brain).
Day 1   O 0 1 2 3 4 5 6
Day 2   O 0 1 2 3 4 5 6
Day 3   O 0 1 2 3 4 5 6
Day 4   O 0 1 2 3 4 5 6
Day 5   O 0 1 2 3 4 5 6

Week 9: Session B-3 (Training with beta, 15 – 18 Hz to improve mood and logical thinking, left and right hemisphere of the brain).
Day 1   O 0 1 2 3 4 5 6
Day 2   O 0 1 2 3 4 5 6
Day 3   O 0 1 2 3 4 5 6
Day 4   O 0 1 2 3 4 5 6
Day 5   O 0 1 2 3 4 5 6

Week 10 : Session B-4 (Training with alpha, beta, and SMR to reduce instability, alternating left and right hemisphere of the brain).
Day 1   O 0 1 2 3 4 5 6
Day 2   O 0 1 2 3 4 5 6
Day 3   O 0 1 2 3 4 5 6
Day 4   O 0 1 2 3 4 5 6
Day 5   O 0 1 2 3 4 5 6

Week 11: Session B-5 (Training with alpha, beta, and SMR to reduce instability, right to left hemisphere of the brain).
Day 1   O 0 1 2 3 4 5 6
Day 2   O 0 1 2 3 4 5 6
Day 3   O 0 1 2 3 4 5 6
Day 4   O 0 1 2 3 4 5 6
Day 5   O 0 1 2 3 4 5 6

Week 12: Session C-2 (SMR 13.5 - 15 Hz).
Day 1   O 0 1 2 3 4 5 6
Day 2   O 0 1 2 3 4 5 6
Day 3   O 0 1 2 3 4 5 6
Day 4   O 0 1 2 3 4 5 6
Day 5   O 0 1 2 3 4 5 6

Congratulations, you've completed 60 consecutive days with the ALERT! Now you can take a break from this program, or continue using it. You're free to do any session that you like. (Perhaps you'd like to try the additional sessions listed below).

Session C-3 (Especially for ADHD and ADD, 30 minutes).
Day 1   O 0 1 2 3 4 5 6
Day 2   O 0 1 2 3 4 5 6
Day 3   O 0 1 2 3 4 5 6
Day 4   O 0 1 2 3 4 5 6
Day 5   O 0 1 2 3 4 5 6

Session C-4 (Depression Reduction, 30 minutes).
Day 1   O 0 1 2 3 4 5 6
Day 2   O 0 1 2 3 4 5 6
Day 3   O 0 1 2 3 4 5 6
Day 4   O 0 1 2 3 4 5 6
Day 5   O 0 1 2 3 4 5 6

Session C-5 (Brain Brightener, 30 minutes).
Day 1   O 0 1 2 3 4 5 6
Day 2   O 0 1 2 3 4 5 6
Day 3   O 0 1 2 3 4 5 6
Day 4   O 0 1 2 3 4 5 6
Day 5   O 0 1 2 3 4 5 6

Session C-6 (Sound Sync— use with music or guided imagery cds).
Day 1   O 0 1 2 3 4 5 6
Day 2   O 0 1 2 3 4 5 6
Day 3   O 0 1 2 3 4 5 6
Day 4   O 0 1 2 3 4 5 6
Day 5   O 0 1 2 3 4 5 6

Session C-1 (Schumann Resonance, 40 minutes).
Day 1   O 0 1 2 3 4 5 6
Day 2   O 0 1 2 3 4 5 6
Day 3   O 0 1 2 3 4 5 6
Day 4   O 0 1 2 3 4 5 6
Day 5   O 0 1 2 3 4 5 6

REFERENCES

Adams, M. (2008). The ADHD scam and the mass drugging of school children. Retrieved on 5/30/2010 from http://www.naturalnews. com/023334_brain_drugs_adhd.html

ADHD Testing (2010). DSM-IV: Formal diagnosis of ADHD. Retrieved on 9/01/10 from http://www.adhdtesting.org/dsm-iv.htm

Adrian, E. & Matthews, B. (1934). The Berger rhythm: Potential dangers from the occipital lobes in man. *Brain,* 57: 355.

Ailtis, J., Ailtis, D. & Bull, M. (2007). Urinary neurotransmitter testing: Myths and misconceptions. *Neuroscience.*

Altman, N. (2007). *The oxygen prescription: The miracle of oxidative therapies.* Rochester, VT: Healing Arts Press.

American Psychiatric Association. (2000). *Diagnostic and statistical manual of mental disorders* (Revised 4th ed). Washington, DC., Author.

American Psychiatric Association. (2002). *Practice guidelines for the treatment of psychiatric disorders.* Washington, DC., Author.

Amen, D. (1999). *Change your brain, change your life: The breakthrough program for conquering anxiety, depression, obsessiveness, anger, and impulsiveness.* New York: Three Rivers Press.

Amen, D. (2002). *Change your brain, change your body: Use your brain to get and keep the body you have always wanted.* New York: Crown / Archetype Books.

Amen, D. (2002). *Healing ADD: The breakthrough program that allows you to see and heal the six types of ADD.* New York: Berkley Trade.

Baker, S. M. (2001). *The circadian prescription: Get in step with your body's natural rhythms to maximize energy, vitality and longevity.* New York: Perigee Trade.

Baughman, F. (1998). Death by ADHD: Who killed Stephanie Hall? Retrieved on 11/14/2010 from http://psychrights.org/Stories/DeathbyADHD.htm

Baughman, F. (2006). *The ADHD fraud: How psychiatry makes patients of normal children.* Bloomington, Indiana: Trafford Publishing.

Beals, G. (1999). Biography of Thomas Edison. Retrieved on 10/19/2009 from http://www.thomasedison.com/biography.html

Block, M. (1996). *No more Ritalin: Treating ADHD without drugs.* Hurst, TX: Kensington Publishers.

Block, M. (2001). *No more ADHD.* Hurst, TX: Block System Publishers.

Block, M. (2010). Psychiatrists are not very happy with me. Breaking free from ADHD. Retrieved on 7/31/2010 from http://blockcenter.com/ADD _ADHD/ Breaking_ Free_ ADHD.html

Bowersox, S.S. & Sterman, M. B. (1981). Changes in sensorimotor sleep spindle activity and seizure susceptibility following somatosensory deafferentation. *Experimental Neurology,* 74:814-828.

Bragin, V. (2007). *How to activate your brain: A practical guide for older adults.* Bloomington, IN: Authorhouse.

Breggin, P. (2001). *Talking back to Ritalin: What doctors aren't telling you about stimulants and ADHD.* Cambridge, MA. Perseus Publishing.

Brookhaven National Laboratory. (2001). New Brookhaven lab study shows how Ritalin works. Retrieved on 10/18/10 from http://www.bnl.gov/bnlweb/pubaf/pr/2001/ bnlpr011501a.html

Brown, S. (2008). Your medical conditions: Is the root your relationships? Institute for Relational Harm Reduction & Public Psychopathy Education.

Retrieved on 11/16/2010 from http://howtospotadangerousman.blogspot.com/2008/05/your-medical-conditions-is-root-your.html

Budzynski, T., Evans, J.R., Abarbanel, A. & Budzynski, H. (2008). *Introduction to quantitative EEG and neurofeedback: Advanced theory and applications.* 2nd Ed., Burlington, MA: Elsevier.

Budzynski, T. H. (1996). Braining brightening: Can neurofeedback improve cognitive process? *Biofeedback*, 24(2), 14-17.

Brain fitness (2008). Arlington, VA: PBS Home Video.

Brain fitness 2: Sight & sound (2009). Arlington, VA: PBS Home Video.

Brain fitness frontiers (2010). Exploring the brain's ability to change throughout life. Arlington, VA: PBS Home Video.

Cannon, W. (1932). *Wisdom of the body.* New York: W. W. Norton and Company, Inc.

Carper, J. (2000). *Your miracle brain.* New York: Harper Collins.

Carnes, A. (1997, November). Schools aren't brick boxes anymore. *Wall Street Journal*, B1, 11/12.

CBS News. (2009). The new drug of choice. Retrieved on 9/5/10 from http://www.cbsnews.com/video/watch/?id=5038367n?source=search_video

Clark, A., Barry, R., McCarthy, R. & Slivovitz, M. (2001). Excess Beta activity in children with ADHD: An atypical electrophysiological group. *Psychiatry Research.* 9/20, 103 (2), 205-218.

Clifton, M. (1998). Hurting and trapping: Teach the children well. Retrieved on 9/9/10 from http://www.sharkonline.org/?P=0000000892

Colbert, D. (2008). *Stress less.* Lake Mary, FL: Siloam / Strang Communications.

CNN News. (1999, May). Six hurt in Georgia high school shooting. Retrieved on 2/23/11 from http://articles.cnn.com/1999-05-20/us/9905_20_conyers.school.shooting.03_1_gunman-students-home-shooting?_s=PM:US

CNS Drug Discoveries. (2006). *CNS drug discoveries: ADHD chapter.* Espicom Business Intelligence Ltd. Retrieved on 7/22/2010 from http://www.researchandmarkets. com/reports/c47133

Cullen, L. (2007). Stress makes you stupid. Work in progress: A daily look at life on the job. Retrieved on 7/14/10 from http://workinprogress.blogs.time.com/2007/08/06/ stress_makes_you_stupid/

Davis, J., Alderson, N., & Welsh. R. (2000). Serotonin and central nervous system fatigue. *American Journal of Clinical Nutrition.* Accessed 1/3/2010 from http://www.ncbi.nlm.nih.gov/pubmed/10919962

DBS (2010). Urinary neurotransmitter testing, not! Retrieved on 11/13/2010 from http://labdbs.com/

DEA (1995). Methylphenidate, A background paper. *National Criminal Justice Reference System.* Abstract, NCJ 166349. Retrieved on 9/4/10 from www.ncjrs.gov/App/publications/abstract.aspx?ID=163349

Demos, J. N. (2005). *Getting started with neurofeedback.* New York: W.W. Norton & Company.

DeNoon, D. (2005). Sudden death in 12 kids on ADHD drug Adderall XR: Sales suspended in Canada. FDA issues U.S. advisory. Retrieved on 9/5/10 from http://www.webmd.com/add-adhd/news/20050210/sudden-death-in-12-kids-on-adhd-drug-adderall

Diamond, M. & Hopson, J. (1999). *The magic trees of the mind.* New York: Penguin Books.

Doidge, N. (2007). *The brain that changes itself: Stories of personal triumph from the frontiers of brain science.* New York. James H. Silberman Books / Penguin.

Dunkle, V. (2010). Psychotropic drugs and failure to warn: Mother's story about the death of her 10-year-old daughter, Shaina, caused by Desipramine toxicity. Retrieved on 9/5/10 from http://www.ritalindeath.com/Desipramine-Death.htm

Éismont, E., Aliyeva, T., Lutsyuk, N. & Pavlenko, V. (2008). EEG correlates of different types of anxiety in 14 to 15 year old teenagers. *Journal of Neurophysiology.* 40 (5-6), 377-384.

Egner, T., Zech, T. F., Gruzelier, J. H. (2004). The effects of neurofeedback training on the spectral topography of the electrocephalgram. *Clinical Neurophysiology.* 115 (11), 2452-60.

FDA Talk Paper T04-60 (2004). New warning for Strattera. Retrieved on 9/5/10 from http://greenmentalhealthcare.com/docs/US_Food_and_Drug_Administration_Warnings_on_ADHD_Drugs.pdf

FDA Advisory Committee. (2005). J & J Concerta psychiatric safety labeling, cardiovascular events are topics for CMTE. Retrieved on 9/5/10 from http://greenmentalhealthcare.com/docs/US_Food_and_Drug_Administration_Warnings_on_ADHD_Drugs.pdf

FDA News Release P07-26. (2007). FDA directs ADHD drug manufacturers to notify patients about cardiovascular adverse events and psychiatric adverse events.

FDA New Release (2005). FDA issues public health advisory on Strattera (Atomoxetine) for Attention Deficit Disorder. Retrieved on 9/5/10 from http://www.fda.gov/ NewsEvents/Newsroom/PressAnnouncements/2005/ucm108493.htm

FDA Public Health Advisory (2005a). Suicidal thinking in children and adolescents being treated with Strattera. Retrieved on 9/5/10 from http://greenmentalhealthcare. com/ docs/US_Food_and_Drug_Administration_Warnings_on_ADHD_Drugs.pdf

FDA Public Health Advisory (2005b). Alert for healthcare professionals Pemoline tablets and chewable tablets (marketed as Cylert).

FDA (2005). Public health advisory: Suicidal thinking in children and adolescents being treated with Strattera (Atomoxetine). Retrieved on 9/5/10 from http://www.fda.gov/ Drugs/DrugSafety/ PostmarketDrugSafetyInformationforPatientsandProviders/ DrugSafetyInformationforHeathcareProfessionals/PublicHealth Advisories/ucm051733.htm

Fernandez, A. & Goldberg, E. (2009). *The sharp brains guide to brain fitness: 18 interviews with scientists, practical advice, and product reviews, to keep your brain sharp.* San Francisco, CA: Sharp Brains, Inc.

Finley, W., Niman, C., Standley, J. & Ender, P. (1976). Frontal EMG biofeedback training of athetoid cerebral palsy patients. *Journal Applied Psychophysiology and Biofeedback.* 1 (2), 169-182.

Fraumeni, P. (2008). The cure for stupid stress. News @ the University of Toronto. Retrieved 7/14/2010 from http://www.news.utoronto.ca/he-said-she-said/the-cure-for-stupid-stress.html

Gevins, A., Smith, M., McEvoy, L. & Yu, D. (1997). High resolution EEG mapping of cortical activation related to working memory: Effects of task difficulty, type of processing, and practice. *Cerebral Cortex Journal.* Vol 7, 374-385.

Gimpel, A. (2007). *Brain exercises to cure ADHD.* Charleston, SC : Book Surge Publishing.

Gottlieb, S. (2001). Therapeutic doses of oral methylphenidate significantly increases extracellular dopamine in the human brain. *British Medical Journal.* Retrieved on 11/12/2010 from http://findarticles.com/p/ articles/mi_m0999 /is_7281_ 322/ai_ 71186032/

Gould, M., Walsh, B., Munfakh, J., et al (2009). Sudden death and use of stimulant medications in youth. *American Journal of Psychiatry.* 166:992-1001. Retrieved 9/5/10 from http://ajp.psychiatryonline.org/cgi/content/ full/166/9/992

Gray, J. & Amen, D. (2003). *The Mars and Venus diet and exercise solution: Create the brain chemistry of health, happiness, and lasting romance.* New York: St. Martin's Press.

Green, A. (1989). Physical and sexual abuse of children. In Kaplan, H. & Sadock, B. (eds). *Comprehensive textbook of psychiatry*, pp. 1962-1970. Baltimore: Williams & Wilkins.

Hall. D. (2001). *Jump start your brain: 50,000 volts of ideas for cranking your cranium and turning your dreams into reality.* Niles, IL: Nightengale Conant.

Hall. W. (2007). *The harm reduction guide to coming off psychiatric drugs.* Northampton, MA: Icarus Project & Freedom Center.

Hasselmoa, M. (2006). The role of acetylcholine in learning and memory. *Current opinion in Neurobiology.* Volume 16 (6), 710-715.

Hebb, D. O. (1949). *The organization of behavior: A neuropsychological theory.* New York: Psychology Press.

Hawley, T. (2000). Starting smart: How early experiences affect brain development. Ounce of prevention fund: Zero to three. Chicago, Illinois.

Herring, J. (2010). ADHD is not a disease. Accessed on 10/4/10 from http://www.totalhealthbreakthroughs.com/2010/03/adhd-is-not-a-disease/

Hill, R. & Castro, E. (2002). *Getting rid of Ritalin: How neurofeedback can successfully treat ADD without drugs.* San Francisco, CA: Hampton Roads Publishing.

Hill, R. & Castro, E. (2009). *Healing young brains: The neurofeedback solution.* San Francisco, CA: Hampton Roads Publishing.

Hinz, M. L. (2010a). Neurotransmitter depletion: The NeuroResearch serotonin and dopamine balanced approach. NeuroResearch Clinics, Inc. Retrieved on 9/3/10 from http://www.neuroassist.com/Neurotransmitter-Depletion-The-NeuroResearch-Serotonin-and-Dopamine-Balanced-Approach.htm.

Hinz, M. L. (2010b). Neurotransmitter depletion. NeuroResearch Clinics, Inc. Retrieved on 9/3/10 from http://www.neuroassist.com/Neurotransmitter-Depletion.htm

Hinz, M. L. (2010c). Neurotransmitter test. NeuroResearch Clinics, Inc. Retrieved on 9/3/10 from http://www.neuroassist.com/neurotransmitter-test.htm

Hoedlmoser, K., Pecherstorfer, T., Gruber, G., et al. (2008). Instrumental conditioning of human SMR (12-15 Hz) and its impact on sleep as well as declarative learning. *Sleep.* 31(10):1401-8.

Indystar (2006). Timeline of incidents: School violence around the world. *Indianapolis Star.* Retrieved 0n 9/9/10 from http://www2.indystar.com/library/factfiles/crime/school_ violence/school_shootings.html

Jainism Global Resource Center (2010). Elephant and the blind men. Retrieved on 11/13/2010 from http://www.jainworld.com/literature/story25.htm

Jensen, E. (2000). *Brain-based learning: The new science of teaching and training.* Thousand Oaks, CA: Corwin Press.

Johnson, J. & Trivitayakhun, P. (2010). Neuroscience and education international conference explores the wonders of the mind and how to keep your child's brain fit to learn. *The Bangkok Post.* Retrieved on 10/10/10 from http://www.bangkokpost.com/life/ education/199727/neuroscience-and-education

Jones, E. (2008). How Could I forgive a killer? *Charlotte Observer.* Retrieved on 11/13/2010 from http://crespifamilyhope.blogspot.com/2010/07/misdiagnosed-mental-illess-drove-david.html

Joyce, M. & Siever, D. (2001). Audio-visual entrainment programs as a treatment for behavior disorders in a school setting. *Journal of Neurotherapy,* 4(2). 9-25.

Kandel, E. (2007). *In search of memory: The emergence of a new science of mind.* New York: W. W. Norton & Company.

Kandel, E., Schwartz, J. & Jessell, T. (2000). *Principles of neural science.* New York: McGraw-Hill Medical.

Kawashima, R. (2004). *Train your brain: 60 days to a better brain.* Teaneck, NJ: Kumon Publishers.

Kawashima, R. (2008). *Train your brain more: 60 days to a better brain.* New York: Penguin Books.

Kuehn, B. (2009). Stimulant use linked to sudden death in children without heart problems. *Journal of the American Medical Association*, 302(6):613-614.

Lantz, D. & Sterman, M.B. (1988). Neuropsychological assessment of subjects with uncontrolled epilepsy: Effects of EEG feedback training. *Epilepsia*, 29(2):163-171.

Law of the Instrument (2010). In Wikipedia. Retrieved 11/13/2010 from http://en.wikipedia.org/wiki/Law_of_the_instrument.

Lee, I. (2008). *Brainwave vibration: Getting back into the rhythm of a happy, healthy life.* Sedona, AZ. Best Life Media.

Levine, B. (2000). *Your body believes every word you say.* Fairfield, CT: Word Works Press.

Lubar, J. (1989). Electroencephalographic biofeedback and neurological applications. *Biofeedback, Principles And Practices For Clinicians.* Baltimore: Williams & Wilkins.

Lubar , J. (1984). Electroencephalographic biofeedback of SMR and beta for treatment of attention deficit disorders in a clinical setting. *Journal of Applied Psychophysiology and Biofeedback*, 9(1), 1-23.

Lubar, J. & Lubar, J. (1984). Electroencephalographic biofeedback of SMR and beta for treatment of attention deficit disorders in a clinical setting. *Biofeedback and Self-Regulation*, 9(1), 1-23.

Lubar , J. (1991). Discourse on the development of EEG diagnostics and biofeedback for attention-deficit/hyperactivity disorders. *Biofeedback and Self-Regulation*, 16 (3).

Lubar, J. & Shouse, M. (1976). EEG and behavioral changes in a hyperactive child concurrent training of the Sensory Motor Rhythm. A preliminary report. *Biofeedback and Self-Regulation*, 1, 293-306.

Lubar , J., Swartwood, M., Swartwood, J. & O'Donnell, P. (1995). Evaluation of the effectiveness of EEG neurofeedback training for ADHD in a clinical setting as measured by changes in T.O.V.A. scores, behavioral ratings, and WISC-R performance. *Biofeedback And Self-Regulation*, 20:83-99. Retrieved on 6/30/2010 from http://www.eegfeedback.org/pdf/o_donnell.pdf

Magnetic Therapy Cure (2010). Schumann Resonance and the scientific work of Dr. Ludwig leads to Electromagnetic Field Therapy. Retrieved on 9/1/10 from http://www.magnetictherapycure.com/Dr_Ludwig.html

Magnetic Therapy Living (2010). Schumann Resonances and your health. Retrieved on 9/2/10 from http://www.magnetic-therapy-living.com/schumann-resonance.html

Mahoney, D. & Restak, R. (1998). *The longevity strategy: How to live to be 100 using the brain-body connection*. New York: John Wiley & Sons, Inc.

Mann, C., Lubar, J., Zimmerman, A., et al. (1991). Quantitative analysis of EEG in boys with ADHD: Controlled study with clinical applications. *Pediatric Neurology*, 8, 30-36.

Miller, G. (2009, July). Gin Miller and 20 years of step aerobics. Interview by Amy Jo MacGowan on Group Fitness Radio. Retrieved on 7/2/2010 from http://www.groupfitness radio.com/fitness-presenters/episode-9-gin-miller-and-twenty-20-years-of-step-aerobics/.

McEwen, B. (2002). *The end of stress as we know it*. Washington, D.C.: Joseph Henry Press. National Academies Press.

McGinty, D. & Sterman, M.B. (1968). Sleep suppression after basal forebrain lesions in the cat. *Science*, 160:1253-1255.

McGinness, D. (1989). ADD: The emperor's new clothes. In Fisher, S. & Greenberg, R. eds. *The limits of biological treatments for psychological distress: Comparisons with psychotherapy and placebo*. New York: Erlbaum Publishers.

McKay, M. & Fanning, P. (1997). *The little book of relaxation and stress reduction: Simple daily practices that can really change your life*. New York: MJF Books / Fine Communications.

Monastra, V.J. (2005). *Parenting children with ADHD: 10 lessons that medicine cannot teach*. Washington, DC: American Psychological Association.

Musca, J. (2009). Drug crimes Florida attorney John Musca discusses evidence between psychiatric meds and violent criminal behavior. Retrieved on 9/9/10 from http://www. floridacriminalattorneysblog. com/2009/07/tom-cruise-v-matt-laurer-in-li.html

Newman, K. (2007). Before the rampage: What can be done? Chronicle Review of Higher Education. Retrieved on 9/9/10 from http://chronicle. com/article/Before-the-Rampage-What-Can/15019

New York Times (1988, October 15). Killer of girl in casino gets life term. Retrieved on 9/9/10 from http://www.nytimes.com/1998/10/15/us/killer-of-girl-in-casino-gets-life-term.html?ref=jeremy_strohmeyer

Norris, S. L., & Currieri, M. (1999). Performance enhancement training through neurofeedback. *Journal of Genetic Psychology, 124*, 311–320.

Oktar, A. (2010). The miracle of hormones: Communication in nerve cells. Retrieved on 08/05/10 from http://www.creationofman.net/ chapter3/chapter3_24.html#64

Parker, S. (1998). *Human body*. New York: DK Publishing.

Patel, F. (2010). The human body is about two-thirds oxygen. Accessed on 11/16/2010 from http://www.oxygen-review.com/human-body.html

Pfurtscheller, G. (2008). Sensorimotor EEG rhythms during execution, imagination and observation of movement. *Clinical Neurophysiology. 119*(1), S23, 91 – 509.

Physicians' desk reference. (64 ed). (2010). Montvale, NJ: Thomson PDR.

Pocket English Idioms (2010). Today's idiom: You can't teach an old dog new tricks. Accessed on 2/1/2011 from http://www.goenglish.com/ Idioms/You+Can%E2%80%99t+Teach+An+Old+Dog+New+Tricks.asp

Pringle, E. (2006). FDA forgot a few ADHD drug related deaths and injuries. Accessed on 2/1/2011 from http://www.lawyersandsettlements. com/articles/00103/adhd_fda.html

Quinn, P.O. & Stern, J.M. (1991). *Putting on the brakes: Young people's guide to understanding ADHD.* New York: Magination Press.

Ratliff, B. (2008). Van Morrison on science, the spiritual and rituals. *New York Times.* Retrieved on 7/10/2010 from http://www.nytimes. com/2008/03/17/arts/music/17van. html

Restak, R. (2002). *Mozart's brain and the fighter pilot: Unleashing your brain's potential.* New York: Three Rivers Press.

Robbins, J. A. (2008). *Symphony in the brain: The evolution of the new brainwave biofeedback.* New York: Grove Press.

Romain, T. & Verdick, E. (2005). *Stress can really get on your nerves.* Minneapolis: Free Spirit Publishing.

Roth, S.R., Sterman, M.B., & Clemente, C.C. (1967). Comparison of EEG correlates of reinforcement, internal inhibition, and sleep. *Electroencephalography and Clinical Neurophysiology*, 23, 509-520.

Rush, C.R. & Baker, R.W. (2001). Behavioral pharmacological similarities between methylphenidate and cocaine in cocaine abusers. *Experimental Clinical Psychopharmacology*: 2-9(1): 59-73. Retrieved on 9/4/10 from www.ncbi.nlm.nih. gov/pubmed/11519636

Satterfield, J. & Dawson, M. (1971). Electrodermal correlates of hyperactivity in children. *Psychophysiology.* 8: 191-197.

Satterfield, J.; Lasser, L.; Saul, R. & Cantwell, D. (1973). EEG aspects in the diagnosis and treatment of Minimal Brain Dysfunction. *Annals of New York Academy of Science.* 2/28; 205: 274-282.

Schumann Resonances (2010). In Wikipedia. Retrieved 11/14/2010 from http://en.wikipedia.org/wiki/Schumann_resonances

Sears, B. (2003). *The Omega Rx zone: The miracle of the new high dose fish oil.* New York: Harper Paperbacks.

Sears, B. (2007). What the brain loves: Adequate blood flow. *American Chiropractor,* 29(2).

Shouse, M.N. & Sterman, M.B. (1979). Changes in seizure susceptibility, sleep time and sleep spindles following thalamic and cerebellar lesions. *Electroencephalography Clinical Neurophysiology.* 46:1-12.

Shouse, M.N. & Sterman, M.B. (1981). Sleep and kindling: Effects of generalized seizure induction. *Experimental Neurology,* 71:563580.

Sightings (2000). Boy apparently dies from long term Ritalin use. Retrieved on 9/5/10 from http://www.rense.com/general/rit.htm

Sinha, G. (2005, July). Training the brain: Cognitive therapy as an alternative to ADHD drugs. *Scientific American.*

Skrzypek, J. (2010, May). Website sells Kip Kinkel letters. KEZI News. Retrieved on 11/16/2010 from http://www2.indystar.com/library/factfiles/crime/school_violence/ school_shootings.html

Sprenger, M. (1999). *Learning and memory: The brain in action.* Alexandria, VA: Association for Supervision & Curriculum Development.

Sprenger, M. (2010). *The leadership brain for dummies.* Indianapolis, IN: For Dummies Books.

Steinberg, M. & Othmer, S. (2004). *ADD: The 20-hour solution: Training minds to concentrate and self-regulate naturally, without medication.* Bandon, OR: Robert D. Reed Publishers.

Sterman, M. B. & Macdonald, L. R. (1978). Effects of central cortical EEG feedback training on incidence of poorly controlled seizures. *Epilepsia,* 19(3):207-222.

Sterman, M. B., Macdonald, L. R. & Stone, R. K. (1974). Biofeedback training of the Sensorimotor EEG rhythm in man: Effects on epilepsy. *Epilepsia*, 15:395-417.

Sterman, M. B., Wyrwicka, W. (1967). EEG correlates of sleep: Evidence for separate forebrain substrates. *Brain Research*, 6, 143-163.

Sterman, M. B., Wyrwicka, W. & Roth, S.R. (1969). Electrophysiological correlates and neural substrates of alimentary behavior in the cat. *Annals of the New York Academy of Sciences*, 157: 723-739.

Sterman, M. B., Goodman, S. J. & Kovalesky, R. A. (1978). Effects of sensorimotor EEG feedback training on seizure susceptibility in the rhesus monkey. *Experimental Neurology*, 62(3):73S-747.

Sterman, M. B. & Kovalesky, R. A. (1979). Anticonvulsant effects of restraint and pyridoxine on hydrazine seizures in the monkey. *Experimental Neurology*, 65:78-86.

Stewart, R. (2010). NeuroWellness natural ADHD program. Retrieved on 11/16/2010 from http://www.neurowellness.com/adhd-program

Stroganova, T., Nygren, G., Tsetlin, M., et al. (2007). Abnormal EEG lateralization in boys with autism. *Clinical Neurophysiology*, 118 (8), 1842-1854.

Swanson, J. M. (1993). Research synthesis of the effects of stimulant medication on children with ADD: A review of reviews. Executive Summary prepared for Division of Innovation and Development, Office of Special Education Programs, Office of Special Education and Rehabilitation Services, U.S. Department of Education. Washington, DC: Chesapeake Institute.

Swanson, J. M. (1993, January 27-29). Medical intervention for children with Attention Deficit Disorder. Proceedings of the Forum on the Education of Children with Attention Deficit Disorder, pp. 27-34. Washington, DC: U.S. Department of Education. Office of Special Education and Rehabilitation Services, and Office of Special Education Programs, Division of Innovation and Development.

Swingle, P. (2008). *Biofeedback for the brain: How neurotherapy effectively treats depression, ADHD, autism and more.* New Brunswick, NJ: Rutgers University Press.

Tansey, M. A. (1984). EEG SMR biofeedback training: Some effects on the neurological precursors of learning disabilities. *International Journal of Psychophysiology*, 3, 85-99.

Tansey, M. (1993). Ten-year stability of EEG biofeedback results for a hyperactive boy who failed the fourth grade perceptually-impaired class. *Biofeedback & Self-Regulation*, 18 (1), 33-38.

Tansey, M. & Bruner, R. (1983). EMG and EEG biofeedback training in the treatment of a 10-year-old hyperactive boy with a developmental reading disorder. *Journal Applied Psychophysiology and Biofeedback*, 8 (1), 25-37.

Thompson, J. D. (2010). Sleep / waking / awakening. Center of Neuroacoustical Research. Retrieved on 7/30/2010 from http://www.neuroacoustic.com/sleep.html

Thompson, L. & Thompson, M.(1998). Neurofeedback combined with training in metacognitive strategies: Effectiveness in students with ADD. *Applied Psychophysiology and Biofeedback*, 23(4).

Turcotte, M. (2010). Foods that increase dopamine and serotonin. Retrieved on 11/16/2010 from http://www.livestrong.com/article/86350-foods-increase-dopamine-serotonin/

Valenstein, E. (2002). *Blaming the brain: The truth About drugs and mental health.* Ann Arbor, MI: Free Press.

Verhovek, S. H. (1999). Teenager to spend life in prison for shootings. *New York Times.* Retrieved on 12/14/08 from http://query.nytimes.com/gst/ fullpage.html?res=9D05E4DA1E3AF932A25752C1A96F958260

Volkow, N., Wang, G., Kollins, S., et al. (2009). Evaluating dopamine reward pathway in ADHD. *Journal of the American Medical Association.* 302 (10), 1084-1091.

Volkow, N., Wang. G., Fowler. J., et al.(2001). Therapeutic doses of oral methylphenidate significantly increases extracellular dopamine in the human brain. *Journal of Neuroscience*, 2001, 21:RC121:1-5. Retrieved on 11/15/2010 from http://www.jneurosci.org/cgi/content/abstract/20014896

Walker, S. (1998). *The hyperactivity hoax*. New York: St. Martin's Press.

Wiedemann, H. (1994). The Pioneers of Pediatric Medicine: Hans Berger. *European Journal of Pediatrics*, 153, 10, 705. Retrieved on 2/23/11 from http://www.springerlink.com/content/q4285240572603q0/

Whalen, C., Henker, B., Collins, B., et al. (1979). A social ecology of hyperactive boys: Medication effects in structured classroom environments. *Journal of Applied Behavior Analysis*. 12, 65-81.

Wise, A. (2002). *Awakening the mind: A guide to harnessing the power of your brainwaves*. New York: Tarcher Books.

Wingert, P. (1996, March). Ritalin: Are we over medicating our kids? *Newsweek*.

Wyrwicka, W. & Sterman, M. B. (1968). Instrumental conditioning of the sensorimotor cortex EEG spindles in the waking cat. *Physiology and Behavior*, Vol. 3, 703–707.

Young, J. G. (1981). Methylphenidate-induced hallucinosis: Case histories and possible mechanisms in action. *Developmental and Behavioral Pediatrics*, 2, 35-38.

RECOMMENDED READING

Amen, D. (2002). *Change your brain, change your body: Use your brain to get and keep the body you have always wanted.* New York: Crown/Archetype Books.

Amen, D. (2002). *Healing ADD: The breakthrough program that allows you to see and heal the six types of ADD.* New York: Berkley Trade.

Amen, D. (1999). *Change your brain, change your life: The breakthrough program for conquering anxiety, depression, obsessiveness, anger, and impulsiveness.* New York: Three Rivers Press.

Bard, A. & Bard, M. *The complete idiot's guide to understanding the brain.* Indianapolis, IN: Alpha Books.

Block, M. (2001). *No more ADHD.* Hurst, TX: Block System Publishers.

Block, M. (1996). *No more Ritalin: Treating ADHD without drugs.* Hurst, TX: Kensington Publishers.

Breggin, P. (2001). *Talking back to Ritalin: What doctors aren't telling you about stimulants and ADHD.* Cambridge, MA. Perseus Publishing.

Doidge, N. (2007). *The brain that changes itself: Stories of personal triumph from the frontiers of brain science.* New York. James H. Silberman Books / Penguin.

Csikszentmihalyi, M. & Jackson, S. (1999). *Flow in sports: The keys to optimal experiences and performances.* Champaign, IL: Human Kinetics.

Gray, J. & Amen, D. (2003). *The Mars and Venus diet and exercise solution: Create the brain chemistry of health, happiness, and lasting romance.* New York: St. Martin's Press.

Hall. D. (2001). *Jump start your brain: 50,000 volts of ideas for cranking your cranium and turning your dreams into reality.* Niles, IL: Nightengale Conant.

Hallowell, E. (2006). *Dare to forgive: The power of letting go and moving on.* Deerfield Beach, FL: HCI Books.

Hill, R. & Castro, E. (2002). *Getting rid of Ritalin: How neurofeedback can successfully treat ADD without drugs.* San Francisco, CA: Hampton Roads Publishing.

Jensen, E. (2000). *Brain-based learning: The new science of teaching and training.* Thousand Oaks, CA: Corwin Press.

Kandel, E., Schwartz, J. & Jessell, T. (2000). *Principles of neural science.* New York: McGraw-Hill Medical.

Newquist, H. P. (2005). *The great brain book: An inside look at the inside of your head.* New York: Scholastic Reference.

Sprenger, M. (1999). *Learning and memory: The brain in action.* Alexandria, VA: Association for Supervision and Curriculum Development.

Swingle, P. (2008). *Biofeedback for the brain: How neurotherapy effectively treats depression, ADHD, autism and more.* New Brunswick, NJ: Rutgers University Press.

Tansey, M. (1993). Ten-year stability of EEG biofeedback results for a hyperactive boy who failed the fourth grade perceptually-impaired class. *Biofeedback & Self-Regulation*, 18 (1), 33-38.

Walker, S. (1998). *The hyperactivity hoax.* New York: St. Martin's Press.

TESTIMONIALS FROM ALERT USERS

"I'm a 33-year-old man with ADD, and have been using your device. Since I found your light and sound machine, I've noticed a pronounced improvement in my ADD:

• I'm out of the house, and on my way to work in 15 minutes, instead of 45 minutes.
• I'm able to remain task-oriented far better.
• I can perform simple tasks such as getting dressed, or doing the dishes, far faster than ever before.
• My frustration levels have dropped significantly.
• I'm not a salesman, or an agent for this company, I'm just a customer who has had a life-changing experience."

Mark Meincke
Alberta, Canada

Better Grades In School

"My son's attitude at home has improved greatly. He is now able to discuss situations rather than fight about them. His marks and behavior in school have improved greatly."

Patty Tucker
Edmonton, Alberta, Canada.

Child Improves Vocabulary

"My child's vocabulary has increased from approximately 15 words to 35 words over a two-week period. For the first time ever, we are able to communicate clearly with him. We have observed many wonderful new things he is now able to do. These are great accomplishments for my son."

Penny Siminiuk
Edmonton, Alberta, Canada.

My Entire Family Uses The ALERT

"My son and I have been using ALERT for 15 days (once a day). We both have ADHD and we are both on medication for several years. Against all expectations, my son has been off medication for five days and it is going really well. Once a month we tried to have him off medication for one day but our trials threw us into despair. Without medication, our son's behavior was very stressful. Medication works well for school and concentration but I worried about his lack of appetite, which is a side effect of the medication. Our son was not putting on normal amount of weight nor growing well. Without the medication, our son was also very agitated and put himself and others in danger. In the evening, once the medication stopped working, he had many rows with us, and I spent my time really stressed out at the thought of "what is he going to do next?" However, after only 15 days with the ALERT, there are significant positive changes. Personally, I also stopped medication for a week. I find the ALERT sessions extremely relaxing and feel refreshed afterwards. Our son and I are really enjoying our daily ALERT sessions and we don't need to be reminded because it is rather pleasurable to slide into this state of deep relaxation. Now, my son is much more centered. Eventually, the whole family wanted to try the device. My husband is working long hours in a very stressful environment. He says it is a fantastic way to relax at work during the lunch break and then go back at full-speed afterwards. Our other two children do not have ADHD but enjoy the ALERT for relaxation. The ALERT seem to work for everyone here, ADHD or not!"

Danielle from Germany

"With the ALERT, my son has made improvements in many areas such as sleep, school, and social skills. We are very happy."

Eileen Hannah
Edmonton, Alberta, Canada.

"My son is sleeping better. He was able to sit through the whole ALERT session and really enjoyed himself!"

Jeannine Hepburn
Edmonton, Alberta, Canada.

"With the ALERT, my son has gone through a dramatic change. He is now much calmer and relaxed. He is progressing very well in school and has gone up the equivalent of three grade point levels. He has settled down a lot. I truly believe this works!"

Karen Hihn
Edmonton, Alberta, Canada.

From F To A+ In School

"My son is much more cooperative now. He recently brought home a mark of 95% in a course that he was failing in just last semester."

Debbie Snatynchuk
Edmonton, Alberta, Canada.

Big Improvement At School & Home

"I just wanted to give you a two-week update on my daughter. She is borderline ADHD. Her teacher started using a checklist for concentration prior to the spring break in March. Before the ALERT, she had a 6 or 7 out of 10 possible checkmarks. After the ALERT, she has had a perfect score every day. At home, my husband and I are finding her much more cooperative, less argumentative and she is doing her homework without bouncing up and down 100 times. I asked the teacher for work to be completed at home today and she has been working on it for the past two hours without complaint! Unbelievable! One of the biggest changes is her attitude towards us. She realizes right away that she stepped over the line and apologizes almost immediately. Her temper outbursts are almost non-existent. My husband also tried a session when he had a headache and his headache went away."

Karen Rodway
Edmonton, Alberta, Canada.

Goodbye To Disorganization, Drugs & Alcohol!

"I want to share a success story with you. It involves my first student study using your light and sound machine. His name is TC, age 19. He had completed his freshman year at college and had significant problems academically. He had been on Wellbutrin and Concerta throughout his freshman year, to no avail. He underachieved badly and had tremendous difficulty getting organized and staying focused. He is an alcohol and drug-free person, so there were no substance abuse issues. Over the summer, I began using the light and sound machine with him. He discontinued his medication with the knowledge and cooperation of his psychiatrist and improved in mood, attitude and behavior over the next eight weeks to the point where his parents purchased a device for him to take back to school and use. Needless to say, he did exceedingly well during his sophomore year, has stayed off the medication, and is now in Italy as a visiting student from his college in New York. When TC returned for a visit at Thanksgiving, he came in to say hello. TC was bright-eyed, focused, engaging, smiling. It was just a joy to behold the newly found confidence he exuded!

Paul Botticell
East Setauket, NY.

A Brilliant Solution For ADHD

"We came across your light and sound machine by accident, but what a Godsend this device has proven to be! Your device proved to be a brilliant solution to help combat ADHD. We have also used the device continuously to relieve stress and bring a calming mood to the staff at Helping Hands UK Org. We fully recommend and applaud the device and would encourage any organizations such as ours to utilize such a device. We cannot recommend this device enough."

Graham J. Hadlington
Helping Hands UK Organization. United Kingdom

"Just a quick note to say thanks for the replacement Omniscreen eyeglasses. It's been working wonders for a number of different problems (insomnia, relaxation, child with ADD). The ALERT is an amazing tool. Again, let me say thank you for replacing the Omniscreen glasses so quickly and for being such nice folks."

Sinead Nulty
Drogheda, Ireland.

ALERT Changed My Child's Future Forever

"My son had a Special Ed teacher who told us he would require learning assistance from grade two to nine due to his inability to read proficiently and his inability to concentrate.

My son exhibited signs of extremely active behavior from a very early age. During kindergarten he received testing and we were informed he showed all of the symptoms of ADHD. My son found the educational system very challenging and his learning to read almost tore our family apart. By the end of grade one, neither my husband nor I would attempt to read with him because he couldn't concentrate long enough to visually recognize the word STAR. He is fascinated with stars, space etc, this simple word frustrated him totally as did words like THE and AND. It also made him really recognize internally for the first time that he was different and that hurt him a lot. What it also did was make him very competitive in other areas of his life, to compensate for the pain and lack of success in the scholastic arena. Of course, this lead to new problems aside from the academic challenges that he was already facing.

"In October 1994, we were fortunate enough to learn about your light and sound machine though a local television show followed by an evening seminar. By this point, we had nothing to lose, as neither my husband nor I believe that the masking of symptoms through the use of medication is a lifetime solution. We had tried a number of things including diet modification with only marginal results, if any. We purchased the audio-visual entrainment (AVE) unit and gave our son a future.

"In early November 1995, I was asked to attend a private meeting at my son's school. The number of people attending was more than at any other previous meeting. From experience, I had learned that bad news seems to take teamwork to deliver, and the worse the news, the bigger the team. Therefore, I was extremely apprehensive, even though my son seemed to be doing better than ever. He was really enjoying school and having real success in all areas, as evidenced by the marks he was achieving in his notebooks and homework assignments.

"At that meeting, I received the second best news in my son's life to date. The first best news was at birth, when I was told by his pediatrician that a birth defect affecting the shape of his skull would in no way impair nor affect his intellectual capabilities. The news was that the school felt that if my son kept up his academic performance for the rest of the school year, he should be removed from the special program. He progressed beyond the program and could function satisfactorily in regular class with only a modified Language Arts program. He was the first person in our county ever to leave the program because he had academically moved beyond it. The reason there were so many people attending the meeting because they wanted to share in this 'first of its kind' success. The moral of this story is that it takes the biggest teams to share great news.

"Well, we're now a year later and my son had his first report card as a student in standard class. His lowest mark was in math, 62%. His teacher says this no way accurately reflects reality, this is his mark in spite of submitting less than half of his fifth grade homework assignments. His highest mark was in Science at 79%. He is now reading at the top end of Grade four level. At the rate he is progressing, I wouldn't be surprised if he is required to follow the standard grade 6 Language Arts Program.

"The report card's comments section was our biggest joy. His teacher wrote that he works well with others, works well in group situations, is cooperative, and fun to have in the class.

"Like many other families, we suffered all of the pain, agony and frustration that a learning impairment entails. Your light and sound machine is giving our son the future we would never have dreamed possible just over two years ago.

"If I had only one wish, it would be that all children who may be symptomatic of ADD or ADHD or any other learning impairment would have the same opportunity to experience this light and sound machine, because every child should have the right to a future. "

Deb St. Jean
Sherwood Park, Alberta, Canada.

Professional Driver Is More Focused With The ALERT

"Wow, it's been two months since I received your light and sound machine and I've been using it every day. I like it. My friends say that I'm calmer, that my hand tremor isn't as noticeable, and neither is my ADD.

The device makes meditation so easy, as I don't have to worry about falling asleep, unless I want to. My creativity has improved. I drive for a living, and feel that I am better focused, thanks to these sessions."

Mark Belisl
Saskatoon, Saskatchewan, Canada.

No More Ritalin For Kindergartner

"Life was a nightmare! It all began when my son was in kindergarten. He was a very happy little boy. We were so excited when he started kindergarten because he was so bright.

"We took him to a pre-kindergarden screening, for everything from speech and hearing to motor skills. The nurses and therapists seemed to be very impressed with David. His skills were good. But then they tested him for things that took a lot of attention. As his mother, I thought that he had done exceptionally well. But the professionals very quickly recommended that my husband and I hold David back from school for one year.

"That's when the nightmare began. At the first parent-teacher conference, David's attention span was not at the level of a six-year-old. He finished the school year, but at the end of kindergarden, the school recommended that David be held back. We refused to sign the paperwork. Then came first grade. The problems got worse. After a while, I finally admitted that David had a problem. Again, the school insisted that David be held back. This time, we agreed.

"David was then tested by the school psychologist. We had known this psychologist for several years, so I trusted his opinion. He very tactfully told us that David might have ADD.

"We went to the doctor, and he prescribed Ritalin, the so-called miracle drug for children with ADD. I began a diary of David's daily activities and moods. Things did not seem to be getting any better. I was still getting daily phone calls from his first grade teacher. So the dosage was increased. Again, no change. Again, the dosage was increased. That's when we started seeing a little change. But again the dosage was increased. At this point David was taking the maximum dosage for a child his size. He began having side effects from the medication. At this point the doctor changed him to Cylert. On a very low dosage, we began seeing what we thought to be miracles.

"David's school work was being completed. He didn't have as much homework. Plus, he was almost back to the normal. For the longest time, we thought we had lost our son. He just wasn't the same on drugs.

"Then the D.A.R.E. Program started at school. This really affected David. He was tired of taking drugs, and he didn't want anyone to know he took anything. They might call him a druggie.

"We went to our doctor and he told us about your light and sound machine. The doctor began doing his very best to get this machine for our son. He also took David off Ritalin.

"After the first ALERT session, there was just a minor change. He could ride all the way home without jabbering. This was approximately a 10-mile ride. We were elated. And, of course, we continued the sessions. We never told his teachers that we were doing anything about David's lack of attention or hyperactivity. We just let it ride. But after each session, we noticed a little more change. The homework was getting done, there was less of it, and David seemed much happier. Even though we were having a crisis at home, David was handling it very well. But in then magical things began to happen. It was like David had bloomed. The homework was down to a minimum, and my husband and I were truly ready for the upcoming parent-teacher conference.

"The teacher started off with 'Has something changed at home? David is doing wonderfully! His homework is complete, his grades are up, and his attention in class is unbelievable!' Of course, I wanted to go hug her. It was the first good conference we had ever had with any of David's teachers. His grades all came up but one. And that was reading. But he did maintain the C that he was carrying. We have continued to see remarkable things happen to David. As a result of the good grades he made it on the Merit Roll. This is not so much for grades as it is for progress.

"As a result of using the ALERT, our son is much easier to live with as a person. There are no more repeated instructions, and no more senseless fights with his little sister. Life is just so much easier now. I couldn't even begin to put into words the relief, the happiness and the thankfulness that the machine has brought to our family.

"In closing, I think any parent with a child who is having problems of any kind, with learning or behavior should be addressed by the machine. Thanks for ending our nightmare and making life just a little bit easier!"

Gwenda Travis
Albuquerque, NM.

Decreased ADHD Drugs By 1/3 With The ALERT

"The more I use your light and sound machine, the more that I like it. My winter blues fade away when I use your device. I used to wake up in a fog and now it's just a joy. I've been singing and humming all day long while I work. After 22 minutes, I feel so calm and serene.

"Besides lifelong ADHD, I have neuropathy in my feet as I also have been living with HIV/AIDS for 23 years, so keeping my stress levels in check is very important.

"I have used many alternative methods to keep my life in balance and still am quite vibrant and alive but this winter has been pretty hard on me and the depression/anxiety was mounting strong. I noticed such a difference in just three days after using your light and sound machine. I decreased my ADD medication by one third with your device and my doctor's supervision."

Kurt Scott
St. Paul, MN.

Dramatic Improvements From Child Expelled From School

"My son, Karl, has always had difficulty concentrating in school. He has been suspended, expelled and transferred from several schools since first grade. However, we have witnessed many encouraging changes in Karl since he began using the light and sound machine. He has become more cooperative at home and at school. I recommend this light and sound machine for anyone suffering from ADD or ADHD. Instead of drugs, try this device first."

Michelle Mackay
Edmonton, Alberta, Canada.

Improved Concentration & No More Fighting At School

"My son has ADHD and as a result has problems concentrating in school. He also got into fights in the schoolyard. I first heard about the light and sound machine on the TV news. He has been using the unit since the end of November and the change in him has been very dramatic. He no longer gets into fights at school, and has a better concentration in the classroom. He is a lot calmer and is able to focus better. His teacher has also noticed a change. He does his work in class, and has very little homework now. The teacher commented to me, 'It's as if he no longer has ADHD.' He is also a lot happier now and does not get as frustrated like he did before using the device. I recommend the ALERT to anyone with ADHD. The results are astonishing! Thanks for all your help with my son."

Diana Bierworth
Sherwood Park, Alberta, Canada.

ABOUT THE AUTHOR

Nicky Vanvalkenburgh wrote this book after experiencing a remarkable transformation with the ALERT brain training program. She has a Master's in journalism from Regent University, and a Bachelor's in psychology from Eastern University. Her background includes ghost-writing books, technical writing, movie reviews, feature and news articles, marketing and public relations, graphic design, web design, and creating computer-based training programs.

Nicky is a Contributing Writer for *Upstate Parent, Low Country Parent* and *Palmetto Parent* magazines, which are published in South Carolina (circ. 250,000). Occasionally, she also writes for the *American Chronicle*.

Nicky is the Director of 20 Minutes to Less Stress.com, which welcomes over 100,000 visitors yearly (from 26 countries) and has been online since 2005. The website sells stress reduction CDs, and offers an *Awaken Your Brainpower* newsletter.

Nicky was born in the Netherlands, and immigrated to America when she was two years old. She grew up speaking Dutch and English at home. She has lived in various parts of Europe (Italy, Belgium, and Holland) for eight years.

Nicky currently lives in South Carolina, with her husband Jim and their two children. In her spare time, Nicky enjoys exercising at the gym, reading books, networking with people, listening to motivational speakers, eating Thai food, drinking herbal tea, and learning all she can about healthy living.

CONTACT INFORMATION

Nicky VanValkenburgh
20 Minutes to Less Stress, LLC.
29 Smokehouse Drive. Simpsonville, SC 29681
(Email) Nicky@TrainYourBrainTransformYourLife.com
(Website) www.TrainYourBrainTransformYourLife.com

ABOUT DAVE SIEVER (Who Wrote The Foreword For This Book)

Dave Siever is the Owner and Director of Mind Alive, Inc., an electronics manufacturing and design company in Alberta, Canada. Mind Alive designs and manufactures various Audio-Visual Entrainment (AVE) devices, including the ALERT.

For the past 20+ years, Dave Siever has been presenting AVE research at the Association of Applied Psychophysiology and Biofeedback (AAPB), the International Society for Neuronal Regulation (ISNR), and the Futurehealth Brain/Mind Conferences. Mind Alive is proud of their reputation as leaders in the AVE industry by providing outstanding knowledge and expertise to customers.

Dave graduated from the Northern Alberta Institute of Technology (NAIT) in 1978 in Telecommunications. In 1980, Dave accepted a position at the University of Alberta, Faculty of Dentistry, as a Design Technologist. Dave conducted research with Dr. Norman Thomas, an internationally recognized specialist in the area of Temporo-Mandibular Dysfunction and myofacial pain. During his employment with the university, Dave developed equipment for the TMJ research laboratory and Educational Psychology department. These devices included TENS stimulators, biofeedback devices, gnatho-dynamometers, signal processing and EMG spectral analysis equipment.

In 1983, Dave began assistant teaching a Dental Physiology course at the University of Alberta. In 1987 and 1988 he taught the graduate year course for Advance Myofacial Pain and TMJ Diagnostic and Treatment Techniques. Dave published a paper with Dr. Norman Thomas on the effects of audio-visual stimulation in the 4th European Congress of Hypnosis in 1987.

From late 1985 to 1987, Dave provided TMJ consulting services to five dentists in the Edmonton area. Over the years, Dave has helped treat approximately 1500 patients with TMJ and MPD. Dave's realization that many TMJ problems were psychologically related prompted him to pursue his interest in biofeedback. This brought about the inception of the original D.A.V.I.D. in the spring of 1984, which was used in the Faculty of Arts to help acting students overcome stage fright.

Through his company, Mind Alive Inc., Dave has continued to develop several AVE, Cranio-Electro Stimulation (CES) and biofeedback devices with each new development responding to the changes in technology and the demands of the marketplace. Dave continues to design new products relating to personal growth and development.

Dave served for many years as the chairperson for the Computer Engineering Advisory Council for the Northern Alberta Institute of Technology (NAIT). He is also a member of ASET, ISNR and AAPB.

Dave travels throughout North America lecturing to dentists, medical groups, biofeedback and neurofeedback professionals, teachers and the general public at various conferences about the use of this technology as an alternative method to improved health, accelerated learning and peace of mind.

ACKNOWLEDGEMENTS

I've spent three years writing and researching this book. That's a long time to spend on a work-in-progress. Let me share with you something that happened to me along the way.

One morning, I was sitting in my car, at a red light. I closed my eyes, and imagined myself holding this book. I couldn't help but smile. How exciting it would be when the pieces all came together. I thought about how I wanted to get this book published. I wanted to explain this drug-free method of brain training in such a way that anyone could understand it. I wanted to make my book exciting and interesting to read. I wanted people with ADHD to catch a vision for the ALERT brain training program. Surely, one day, I could help people train their brain and transform their lives. Someday, all of this time and effort that I was investing in my book would be worthwhile.

So, I'm sitting there at the red light, smiling, with my eyes closed. I'm imagining myself holding this book. All of a sudden, I'm interrupted by this knocking sound. It startled me, and I opened my eyes. It was a man in the passenger seat of the car next to me. He was knocking on his car window, and motioned for me to roll down my window. He was dressed in a business suit, and appeared to be carpooling to work.

The man yelled out to me, "Hey lady, whatcha thinking about, 'cause I sure could use a little bit of happiness right now!"

Whoa, a complete stranger! He seemed nice enough, with a big smile on his face. Surely, it would be safe to talk to him for a few seconds while watching for the light to change.

"Heh, I'm writing a book... and I was just daydreaming about it being published," I said.

"That's gonna be some book," he yelled back. We were both smiling when the light switched to green. He gave me a thumbs up, and drove off.

It was an interesting encounter. Somehow, that man picked up on my energy and enthusiasm for this book. He called it "a little bit of happiness". Funny how he made an effort to talk to me, perhaps out of curiosity. He was a complete stranger, but he gave me a thumbs up. It was the little bit of motivation that I needed to push forward and finish writing my book.

Sometimes, it's the little things that make all the difference. I'd like to thank my friends and family for helping me on my journey. I'm grateful for my book coach and mentor, Kalinda Rose Stevenson. When I initially wrote about my experience with Ritalin, I just cringed. I was embarassed to tell my story. However, Kalinda assured me that everyone makes mistakes. What matters is that I learned something from my mistakes. If my readers would be encouraged or inspired by reading my story, that's what really matters. Kalinda also encouraged me to have a main point (or thesis) for each chapter, and suggested that I re-write the chapters that didn't make sense. Re-writing was frustrating at times, but now I'm glad that I did. Kalinda also encouraged me to let my personality shine through, and to share personal experiences to make my writing more compelling and persuasive. She also helped me to recognize the importance of this book's message. I'm blessed by Kalinda's coaching, plus her knowledge of writing, storytelling, psychology, persuasion, and rhetoric. Kalinda is always my advocate, and she teaches me perseverance and optimism, which are reflected in this book.

I'm also appreciative of David Siever at Mind Alive, Inc. in Edmonton, Alberta, Canada. He invested his time to make sure that this book was technically accurate. He read at least three drafts of this book, and also asked his psychology intern, Amanda Jackson, to check it for APA Style. Thank you Dave and Amanda, for your help.

I'm grateful to friends and family members who also proofread and offered feedback, including Petrie Ockeloen, Lisette Ockeloen, Daria Cronic, Ken Herman, Michael Landgraf, Jenny Weathers, Mitch Jamison, Lynette Froehlich, Harlan Goerger, and Angela Mckelvey.

A special word of thanks to the folks who wrote endorsements and testimonials for this book and the ALERT brain training system, including Daria T. Cronic, Kenneth Herman, Rita Wiggs, Michael Landgraf, Deborah Merlin, Vincent Harris, Jaime Rohadfox, Harlan Goerger, Lynette Froehlich, Dave Weiner, Kalinda Rose Stevenson, Beau

Garraud, Mitch Jamison, Earma Brown, Lisa Hardwick, Lisette Ockeloen, Michelle Matteson, Caron Goode, Michael Hutchison, Laurie Runyan, Mark Meincke, Patty Tucker, Penny Siminiuk, Danielle, Eileen Hannah, Jeannine Hepburn, Karen Hihn, Debbie Snatynchuk, Karen Rodway, Paul Botticell, Graham J. Hadlington, Sinead Nulty, Deb St. Jean, Mark Belisl, Gwenda Travis, Kurt Scott, Michelle Mackay, and Diana Bierworth.

I'm grateful to the Greenville County Library System, especially the Simpsonville-Hendricks Branch. They're always cheerful about my requests for books and journal articles. They ordered many items for me on Interlibrary Loan. I'll never forget the time they got me a medical textbook on the brain, *Principles of Neural Science* (2000). I thought that I'd have to order it on Amazon, and shell out a hundred bucks! It was exciting to read that book, and discover what medical students are learning in their introductory neuroscience classes. Thank you, librarians at the Hendricks Library in Simpsonville, SC.

As always, I'm fortunate to have the ongoing support and reassurance of my husband, Jim, and our sons, Sean and Perry. I'm also grateful for the inspiration that I receive from my parents, Jan and Petrie Ockeloen, and my in-laws, Cap and Louise VanValkenburgh.

I'd like to send warm wishes to my extended family, Hanneke and Steve Counts; John and Andrew Counts; David and Susan VanValkenburgh; Jake, Josh and Matthew VanValkenburgh; Barbie and Rob Mason; Abby Mason; Mayre and Bill Favaloro; Linda and Jeff Becklund; Robbie and Michelle Castle; Albert Castle; Charles and Jane Downing; and others.

I also send warm wishes to my Dutch relatives: Bert and Janneke Ockeloen, Manda and Martin Swart; Agnes and Jan Meijer; Sonja and Han Si Dihan Ho; Monika and Just Herder; Ilona and Redmer VanLeeuwen; Hans and Loes Esseveld; Josje and Frits Besselink; Marleen Esseveld; Robbert and Henriette Hilhorst; Joop Meinen and Ine Rouwers; Live and Marta Schuster; Astrid Schuster-Mackey; Diana Schuster-Schmitt; Fiona Schuster, and others.

I'm grateful for the support of my friend Angela Toplovich, Director of Bridge to Wellness, LLC. in Simpsonville, SC. Her business offers Colon Hydrotherapy, Thermotherapy (with the Bio-Mat), Ear Candling, and Ionic Footbath. Check out her website at www.YourBridge2Wellness.com

I'd like to give a "shout out" to my group fitness teachers at Sportsclub in Greenville, SC. Most of them aren't aware of this book, but attending their classes always motivates me. Nothing like exercising to the point of exhaustion, to help me think clearly and come to grips with ideas for my writing. Best wishes to Janet Rivett, Gretchen Jacobs, Lynette Froehlich, Jesse Hamlin, Darren Rambo, Kurt Huey, Yvonne Vignjevic, Lee Jackson, Adonia Ray, Laurie Greenway, Amy Farmer, Dina King, Lori Morris, Pam Kavulic, Barbara Seale, Athena Seay, and Angel Irby. Check out the company website at www.Sportsclubsc.com

I'd also like to give a "shout out" to the Imagine Center in Greenville, SC. My teachers and friends include Lee Dillingham, Jaime & Terrie Smith, Jesse Mikell, Stephanie Craig, Jillian Wells, Tina Pressley, and Anna Briggs. Check out their website at www.ImagineCenter.com

I'm grateful for my Facebook friends, who have encouraged me while writing this book: Alan Weissman, Alice Kendall, Alice Lovette, Allison Pittman MacMillan, Andrea Schroen-Martins, Andrew Reinholz, Angela Mckelvey, Anissa Runde, Art & Ann Hannah, Anna Briggs, Anthony Southby, Ashton Benninghoven, Becky Johnson, Bobbie Christmas, Bobby Minor, Bonnie Thoennes Conforti, Brenda Eileen Brack, Brenda Fuller, Brenda Garrison Bilcher, Brenda Tingstrom, Carol Mathers, Caroline Kirkley Taylor, Carolyn Perry, Carrie Creech, Cathi Denman-Elder, Cee Mathers, Chili Nut, Chris Smith, Chris Worthy, Christy Luberger Barajas, Cindi Skinner Rhodes, Cindy Foster Schultz, Cindy Skelton, Clancy Smith, Coney Egar, Crystal Selfridge, Curt Hucks, Cy Selfridge, Dannette Foglesong Shafer. Darcy Wozney Downing, Dave Lakhani, Dawn Applegate, Dawn Ward, Dean Forrest, Deb Small, Debbie Norman Parnell, Debbie Parsons Whitt, Deborah Reinauer Merlin, Deena Medlin, Deirdre Jenkins Hunt, Denissa Lamprecht, Donna & Jose Gutierrez, Earl Henslin, Earma Brown, Elsom Eldridge Jr., Elysia Devost Knudson, Erin Werner, Felicia Armes, George Holcombe, Georgetta Ruth Belch, Gillian Hervey Hayward, Grace Ruffner Lamprecht, Greg Tedder, Hajni Blasko, Harlan Goerger, Holly Harris Smith, Jaime L Rohadfox, Jane Downing. Jane Van Pinxten Mangum, Janet Graziano, Jeanne Witzke, Jen Hall, Jennifer Torres Smith, Jenny Weathers, Jeremy M. Scott, Jess Kennedy Williams, Jesse Hamlin, Jill Crosby, Jimmy Snow, Joanke Nicole Hilhorst, Joe & Marlene Shaw, Joelle Gwynn, John Dawson, John F. Ingrassia, Jonathan Fowler, Jose Carlos Naranjo, Josephine Forrester, Judy M. Graybill, Judy Roberts Wallace,

Julia Sermons Hoyle, Julie VanValkenburgh, Karen Campbell Herrick, Kathleen Terry, Kathy Morris Cassidy, Katie Shafer, Katrina Everett Bianchi, Ken & Erika Griffiths., Ken Owens, Kendall Milburn Delorenzi, Kenny Warfield, Kimberly Smith, Kimberly Ussher, Kimberly Watson Hix, Kita Szpak, Kris Zeke Ward, Kristi Carden, Lancy Pinto, Laura Chandler Blackwelder, Laura-Faye Weir, Laurie Runyan, Lee Dillingham, Lemon Lao, Libby Morse, Lillian Cauldwell, Linda Dara, Linda Reedy Warfield, Lisette Ockeloen, Lois Mae Byrd, Lynda Moldrem, Lynn Emmons, Mandee Glenn, Maran Banta, Marie Sellers, Mark Carpenter, Marlene Joy Shaw, Marnix Groet, Maro Rostom Yacu, Martha Hautala Lindsey, Marybeth Ols Smith, Marylee Decker, Matresia Sullivan, Matthew Huston, Matthew Zhou, Melanie Floyd Hutchinson, Melissa Gilstrap Fowler, Melissa Thomas Ancell, Michael Hutchison, Michael Landgraf, Michael Seriosa, Michele Smith-Hockett, Michelle Matteson, Michiel Ockeloen, Mitch Jamison, Mitchell A. Blass, Molly Rebekah Warren, MonaLisa Smiles, Monique MacKinnon, Monnie Whitson, Nancy Siever, Nannie Krenek, Neva Hanson, Nima Buva, No Ni Man, Obi Bob Efurd, Oliver Riebe, Parker Gutierrez, Pat Clark Millett, Patty Nowell-Odom, Paulyn Glenn, Pete Martin, Peter Van, Pmore Anyas, Randall & Laura Owens, Reena Baranan, Rena Selph Caldwell, Rhonda Edgar Lowder, Rick Johnson, Rita Allen Oliveira, Rita Wiggs, Ritsuko Yano, Robert Ellis, Robert Ockeloen, Robert Reuter, Rob Duffield, Robert Wiggs, Ron Ash, Rosealee Griffiths, Ryan Yow, Sandra & Steve McNulty, Sarah Martin, Sarah Thurston, Sebastiaan Van Wessem, Sharon Rogers-Boyles, Shauna Faye, Shawn Wiederin, Shelly Yohn, Sheri McCune, Sherri L Emmons, Sheryl Renee Duckett, Starlyn Conklin, Stephanie Rivers Luberger, Susan Clark, Susan Steed, Teppi Alexander, Thomas Moore, Tracey Smith Lehman, Tracy Garcia, Travis Shafer, Valeria Sottili, Vernon Wayne Buchanan Jr.,Vicky Odom McClain,Vince Harris, Vonda Skinner Skelton, Walter & Britty Groet, Wanda Hamilton, and Wayne Vandenlangenberg.

Lastly, I thank God for this opportunity (Phillipians 4:13). He gave me a vision for this book, and enabled me to write it. He has provided me with more than I could ever imagine. God has surrounded me with people who care about me. God has given me family and friends who bless me everyday with kind words and actions. They lift me up and make my spirit soar. I'm grateful for all the blessings in my life.

9 780615 297941